NURSE!

NURSE!

a memoir

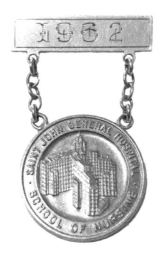

Francene Cosman

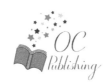

OC
Publishing

Cover and interior book design by
David W. Edelstein

Published by

Halifax, NS
info@ocpublishing.ca
www.ocpublishing.ca

ISBN 978-1-989833-30-8 - Paperback
ISBN 978-1-989833-31-5 - eBook

TO NURSES EVERYWHERE!

Introduction

TIME BENDS MEMORY, LIKE MUSIC FORGOTTEN from the past, until one day a few notes resurface, and the melody returns. In the half century since my student days, certain things remain bright and vivid, untarnished by the passage of time. I came of age in the grip of a hospital, molded by the events described in this memoir. This is my story.

In 1931, the Saint John General Hospital was rebuilt on the former site of a decrepit wooden structure that had passed its best-before date by decades. The new yellow brick building was in its final stage of construction but not yet ready for its official opening. Dr. Arthur Chesley was chosen as the first doctor for the new health centre, and his leadership guided every future operational decision.

Behind the new building stood a wooden annex

that continued to serve as a wing for contagious and infectious diseases. The worst cases were isolated here, and the nurses were constantly putting themselves at risk. This was an age where there were no antibiotics. One can imagine that the nurses' hands were scrubbed raw with carbolic soap in an effort to stay free of disease.

My nursing career had its genesis in 1949 when I was eight years old. It all started with a trip to the Saint John General Hospital that left quite an impression on my young mind.

My mother intended to visit a sick friend, and I was going with her.

"Get your coat on, we're going to the hospital."

At first, I resisted, wondering if someone was going to stick a needle in my arm. We normally had vaccines at school, but my fear was that I would be having one at the hospital that day. My moment of indecision ended as Mother yanked me to the closet and forced me to pull on my coat. We lived on Wentworth Street in the middle of the slums, close enough to the General that we could walk. We took off at a brisk pace. Mother wanted to get there before the visiting hour started.

We pushed the heavy glass and brass doors open and entered the large baronial hall. Visitors were detained here until the precise moment of the evening visit. The one commissionaire on duty stood with his arms crossed, a man not to be questioned. With his chest pushed out, he looked very important. It was his job to announce to visitors the precise moment when they were allowed to go up to the floors—not one minute early and never one minute late!

The waiting area was quiet but expectant with the uneasy talk of family members. Their hushed tones reflected the serious fact that they were here, in a hospital.

The chairs were massive but few, built of heavy oak with carved high backs and leather seats. They were uncomfortable at best, and as a child, taking a brief turn to sit down, my legs and feet swung free. There was an established social order around who could sit. Men took off their hats or caps and sat only if feeble and frail. Chivalry prevailed, so a gentleman would give up his seat to a woman and she in turn permitted a child a moment's rest, then the child got up quickly for another person—a form of musical chairs without the music.

The high ceiling amazed me.

"Is this a church, Mommy?"

She ignored me.

The mahogany panelled walls were hung with beautiful large framed portraits looking down on the visitors.

"Can they see me, Mommy?" I looked up and

painted eyes seemed to stare back. Still no answer from my mom, but this wasn't unusual.

The waiting area became increasingly crowded as the minute hand of the tall mahogany grandfather clock crept closer to 7:00 p.m.

"Visiting time is now open!" the commissionaire's voice boomed.

Everyone in the waiting area made a mad dash for the stairs and elevators. En masse, the horde made its way. With only one brief hour allowed, the full day's worth of catching up had to be compressed.

A marble staircase led to the second-floor landing where the elevators opened and closed. They looked like metal cages with an outer door that drew across like an accordion and closed with a clang.

A shiny brass banister tempted me to run up the stairs and slide down, but hauled along in the grip of my mother's hand, I dared not! Underneath the banister were bronze animals and strange-looking fish, placed so that no one could fall through the space. We squeezed inside the elevator, and once it was full of passengers, the solid door closed silently. It did not feel safe as it bumped and vibrated along its upward path.

"Is it a cage? Are there lions?" This at least caused my mother to glance at me. "What stinks, Mommy?"

She still didn't answer but others around me smiled at my remark as the scent of ether wafted down the elevator shafts from the seventh-floor operating theatres.

As passengers got off at each floor, a whoosh of smelly air came through the open doors. The atmosphere held a mixture of bodily odours from illness and the ever-present disinfectant that was used on all surfaces. The smell stuck in my nose.

"It still stinks, Mommy." I don't remember if I ever had an answer as to the cause.

Shortly after this visit to the hospital, my family left Saint John and moved a few miles away to the village of Renforth. Dad had purchased us a house, a brand new two-storey wood structure with an identical house next to it. Although we mainly had wooden crates that originally held oranges for furniture, we would now have our first secure home. There was a mud yard, later to be seeded, but for now brown and rocky.

My dad was a recovering alcoholic, a violent man in the past, but he had become a member of Alcoholics Anonymous (AA). His transformation resulted in a newly sober father. AA had a prayer that we recited daily: "God grant me the courage to change the things I can, the serenity to accept the things I cannot, and the wisdom to know the difference." That prayer and my father's black leather Bible became the foundation of our new life.

When we first arrived at the new house, my parents, my sister, and I removed our shoes and walked inside. I had never seen shining hardwood floors.

"Why do we have two living rooms, Daddy?"

"It's a dining room."

I was supposed to know what that meant. Alongside the dining room was the kitchen with simple painted wood cupboards and a drop-down ironing board hidden in the wall. A huge pullout bin held fifty pounds of flour that would be well used by my mother, who liked to bake.

I yelled to my sister, "Shirley, come on, hurry up. Let's go upstairs." We found a wide hallway with cupboards for linen, a bathroom, and three bedrooms. Never had I imagined a home of our own, let alone my own bedroom. My sis and I had always shared a bed, covered in old tablecloths for bedding, and now we would separate to our own rooms.

Sis chose the second-largest bedroom with two clothes closets, and I got the smallest with a single closet. My room looked out over the backyard, but from the hall window I could see a forest of trees and long slabs of granite snaking along the earth like so many extended grey centipedes. Nearby was a farm with black-and-white cows.

I ran down the stairs, went out the door in a

flash, and began to explore what I had seen from the upstairs window. I had never been in the woods or a park. The rich scent beckoned me, and a variety of trees with their needles and leaves could not be resisted. The forest was magic. I named it Wonderland.

Moving from a slum with a brothel across the street to the sanctuary of Renforth opened future possibilities for regular attendance at a school, and friends. It sparked my eager, exploring mind. I would have goals, ambition, and a fierce drive to succeed that had lain dormant but now emerged as I left behind the years of hardship.

Chapter 1

SOME PEOPLE ARE BORN TO SING. I WAS BORN TO nurse, but I didn't know it yet.

It would be a weird kid who, when growing up, thought about the future. I wasn't weird.

However, growing up happens, whether wanted or not, and in my eighteenth year, in 1959, choices had to be made. There were few career options for young women. Post-secondary schooling was generally limited to teacher's college, nursing, or secretarial school. If you were lucky enough to have wealthy parents, there were more choices. I didn't have wealthy parents.

As a young girl, I had been inspired by our family doctor, George Bate. When our paths first crossed, I was lying in bed with a high fever, and he, making house calls, was building his country practice. His kind, calm, and knowledgeable demeanour impressed me.

I had ambition and sent an application to Boston University for their pre-med program.

I discussed it with my parents. Neither had a high school education, let alone university. So truly, what could I expect? Eventually, my dad and I had a short chat about my future.

He looked frustrated and that meant he was angry. His eyes shot sparks at me as he asked, "What do you need an education for? You'll get pregnant, get married, and that will be that."

I'm not sure whether he meant it in that order, but it was how it came out. It was my turn to feel angry, and my innards tied up in a knot. I was aware of the growth of the feminist movement in the 1950s, and this was fuelling my desire to have a career and something different from my mother's life of homemaker and servant to my dad.

"Oh shit, Dad, is that how you really think? That I'll get pregnant? Do you think I'm that stupid? I'll never be a mother, ever! And I sure as hell don't plan on staying at home to look after someone's dirty clothes or be a slave!"

I stomped up the stairs, threw myself across the bed, and tried to hold back my rage. Then the tears came. Dad and I were on very different wavelengths when it came to my hopes and what I wanted as a young woman growing up in a decade of change.

Despite a steady stream of dates and a boyfriend,

I didn't have, nor did I want, marriage prospects. I loved to learn new things, liked a good challenge, and wanted more for myself. But my choices were limited. My sister had become a secretary, so naturally, I wanted something different. Teaching, with the summer off, was attractive to me, yet there was no money for college tuition.

Nursing was the closest thing to medicine, so my choice was made by default. I don't recall ever having a serious talk with my parents about my suitability to become a nursing student. Three other high school classmates also decided on this, so I knew I wouldn't be among strangers. It was time to put my parents in the picture.

"Mom, Dad, I'm going to apply to the nursing program at the General. I'll need your help with the cost of the uniforms and some spending money each month, but the room and board will be free."

Truthfully, I think they wanted me off their hands at some point soon, and they were relieved I was taking that route.

The General provided a stipend to each student. This had to offset the cost of sundry items and meet the needs of daily living. It seemed like a bad joke that this amount had not changed since January 1891.

In Victorian times, a first-year student was paid six dollars a month. In the second year, it increased to eight dollars. When the third year of nursing was added to the program in January 1891, the stipend went up to ten dollars. Had this kept pace with inflation, it would have been worth a few hundred dollars by the time I entered the school. But the stipend remained at ten dollars.

To give my dad credit, he offered me fifty dollars a month, and I took it. But I didn't understand the sacrifice it meant.

I had graduated from Rothesay Regional High School in June 1959 with excellent marks, with only one exception—physics. I sent my letter of application to Miss Stephenson, the director of the Saint John General Hospital School of Nursing, accompanied by my school marks and the provincial matriculation results. The "matric," as it was known, was the education standard each student had to achieve to graduate. All students in New Brunswick wrote a common set of exams, not influenced by which school they had attended. I included a character reference from my church minister, the Reverend J. J. Hoyt.

The secretary called my home and asked me to come in to the General and have a preliminary interview with Miss Stephenson, and we set the date and time for the following week. The day of my appointment, I dressed carefully in a pale green linen suit, accessorized by fashionable shoes, gloves, and a purse. I believed in making a good first impression.

I had diarrhea before I even got to Saint John. My bowels were all nerves. The thought of the meeting scared me, and I loaded up on Pepto-Bismol in an effort to quell the churning. My mother drove me to the hospital.

What if she doesn't like me? This negative thought stuck with me as I walked down the long corridor to Miss Stephenson's office, met the secretary, and then, for no apparent reason, was made to wait. When at last I was ushered into the inner sanctum, my mouth was dry, my hands shook, and my armpits were wet.

Miss Stephenson looked me up and down, and I stuck out my hand to give hers a shake. I grabbed it in an enthusiastic, bone-crushing grip and felt her fine, thin fingers crunch in mine.

"How do you do, Miss McCarthy?"

Was that a grimace that flitted across her face? She sat, erect and intimidating, behind a large mahogany desk on a hard wooden chair. Her uniform was so starched it looked like a white cardboard tube. She exuded authority. The green desk lamp cast long shadows on the wall behind her and played its light across her stern features. Her mouth was a thin red line; the lipstick, her only makeup, worsened narrow lip lines. She looked formidable.

"Tell me why you want to be a nurse."

Jeez, I couldn't tell her the truth, that nursing was

a default decision. My mouth ran out of spit, and my words came out half glued to my tongue.

"I want to help people, to heal people who are in pain, to take care of . . ." The thoughts petered out as I realized that she wasn't listening. She was looking at my transcript. I had placed third in my class, but she noted my one low mark.

"You didn't do well in the subject of physics. You'll have a lot of science-based studies in your classes." Then she glanced at my shoulder-length hair and said, "Hair must be short, Miss McCarthy. It cannot touch the uniform collar. Perhaps you should get it cut?"

Was that an order?

"That's all for now, Miss McCarthy. You'll receive a letter from the administration if you are successful. We have many interviews, and we will only accept the very finest of students."

Her emphasis on "the very finest" made me wonder, *Did she view me as fine?* I thanked her and left the office, not sure how I had done but glad it was over. My high heels clicked their way over the heavily waxed floors while my nose detected the ether fumes wafting down the elevator shafts from several floors above. A jittery fear struck my mind. *What will I do if I don't get accepted?* I had no intention of cutting my hair until I knew whether or not I was to be among the new cohort of first-year nursing students.

And then I waited. This was my last carefree summer to swim, play tennis, date, dance, go to corn boils on the shores of the Kennebecasis River, see my friends, and goof off before the hard work began. No responsibility for two precious months. The summer stretched out before me, full of laughter and silliness, which marked the end of my youth. None of us truly knew what lay ahead.

Finally, the day came when an important letter from the Saint John General Hospital arrived. This was a make-or-break moment for my future. I was alone at home and walked to my bedroom to read it. I glanced at the childish decor of my room: stuffed animals, books, magazines, makeup on a tray, and a lot of junk. My hands shook as I ripped open the envelope and read the contents. It advised that I was accepted into the School of Nursing and included a list of what uniforms to order, how to measure for them, and a long, detailed, itemized inventory.

It also stated, "Your time will be spent in uniform or a housecoat, so you will not need as many clothes as you have previously."

"I'M IN!" I screeched, then I ran to the phone and called my best friend.

"Jane! I got my acceptance letter! I'm in! Come over and let's celebrate!"

I glanced at the uniform order and the specifics. Was it a typo or did it really say that the apron's hem must be thirteen inches from the floor? How archaic. The order would consist of aprons, bibs, collars, an engraved pair of nursing scissors, and a traditional navy-blue wool cape that buttoned at the collar.

We were required to wear black leather oxfords, locally sourced at Scovil's, the old-fashioned department store on King Street in Saint John, where the entire interior was a golden oak. We needed black stockings to match the shoes, and since pantyhose didn't exist, they were held up by a garter belt with clips, dangling by elastics, that attached to the top.

It's not possible to look glamourous in a plain black leather shoe with a short, stumpy, rubberized military heel, tied up with laces and worn with matching stockings. Black shoes were the standard for two years until we received our "whites" at the beginning of our third year.

My dad sent off a cheque for the uniforms to the Blandon Company in Montreal. A few weeks later I received a notice from the local post office that a large box was being held in my name.

The tiny post office was a relic from decades past. It had formerly been an outbuilding at the rear of a luxurious summer home on the Kennebecasis River.

When the rail line came along it cut the property in half. Each time a train passed by, all talking stopped inside as the building shook on its foundation. Now, a highway passed its door. The wood clapboard shingles were weathered, darkened, and flaking with age.

The postmaster, Mr. Fitzgerald, better known as Fitzie, could be described in a similar manner. A veteran of the Great War, he always sported a navy-blue blazer over grey trousers. He worked at the desk of the stamp section, inside a glass cubicle. He conducted his business in a stern, professional manner. Most folks knew Fitzie, and the decrepit building, with its slight lean, was the local centre for chat.

As I drove to the office, memories flooded my mind. I had been a juvenile stamp collector, and it was from Fitzie that I purchased first-day covers of new Canadian stamps and special commemoratives. When they arrived, he always called me at home; his voice was recognizable—shaky and frail. That he took an interest in me was surprising.

"Miss McCarthy? I think you should come in and see the new issues. I'm sure they'll interest you." Fitzie always told me whenever something special was happening in the philatelic world. I had bought a full sheet of stamps celebrating the Queen's coronation.

The tiny building also housed a vast array of penny candy, enjoyed by children for decades. Three pieces for a penny was a good deal. Stepping through the doorway, my sense of smell went on high alert. My nose twitched, and I tasted the chocolate before it ever left the display jar and entered my watering mouth. I ate my fill of candy. I would load up a brown paper bag of mixed jujubes, mint leaves, fudge squares, licorice, and Ganong marshmallow-filled, chocolate-coated candy. Sometimes cheating, I stuck an extra piece in the bag. The larger ones went for two for a penny, and some whoppers went for a penny each. For twenty-five cents I could nibble my way through seventy-five candies in a brown paper bag on my way home from school.

But back to the business of picking up my package!

The loose gravel at the shoulder of the road in front of the post office left little room for a car to pull alongside, and a blind knoll at the top of the hill made it a precarious stopping spot. The large, heavy box from Blandon's took up most of Fitzie's interior cubicle space. Forgetting his age, Mr. Fitzgerald offered to help me place my package in the trunk of the car. We picked it up, struggled through the single door, and hefted it into the rear of the car. Excited, with butterflies in my tummy, I raced home.

I cut into the cardboard box with a large kitchen knife, ripped open the packing tissue, and uncovered the blue-and-white pinstripe uniform, the aprons and bibs, a man's hanky, and a small packet containing my nursing scissors engraved with my name. The heavy wool nurse's cape rested at the bottom. The contents were a folded, wrinkled mess smelling of the factory, but I couldn't wait to try them on. The hospital laundry would soon turn them into starched perfection.

I took the stairs to my bedroom two at a time with the uniform in my arms, then stripped down and tried on all the items. When I glanced in the mirror, I felt a tingle of surprise. Looking back at me was a young woman who had matured by simply donning a uniform.

Hey! I look like a nurse!

I called my friend Jane. "Oh my gosh, you've got to see this! Bike over, hurry . . . I'm so happy."

We took pictures of the two of us standing on my front lawn. The apron was long, meeting the requirement of thirteen inches above the floor. But it enhanced my tiny waist, so that was a plus. Although the bib hid any aspect of the female torso, it was designed to keep the pinstriped dress clean from the inevitable contaminants of the nursing ward.

The nurse's cap was a plain white hanky. The cap wasn't required until, as a new student, I passed the probationary period. It would take five months before we even knew if we would earn the right to wear it. By then, all seventy-six students should have learned how to make up the starch-sugar soak, dip the hanky into the goo, and then press it onto the side of a fridge. Every starch wrinkle had to be fingered out. Eventually, it all hardened and would be peeled off the fridge and folded in a special manner. Voila! A nurse's cap held together with straight pins. If you accidentally stuck a pin into your finger and splodged blood onto the fabric, it was back to the wash basin to start all over.

Packing my suitcase to leave home for the first time caused mixed emotions. The tiny bedroom that became mine at age eight held the remnants of my preteen years tucked into the back of a closet. I was fourteen when my sis left home and I took over her larger room with its two closets, an unusual feature in a home built in the early 1950s. Every time a summer storm came through, with walloping winds and thunder, my mom and I would gather in the safety of the walk-in closet and shriek in fear of a lightning strike. Perhaps we should have tossed out the metal cans of tennis balls and the battered rackets. My bedroom was my refuge. It held memories of laughter and tears.

I looked around my room at the toy animal collection. My bookcase-style bed held all my *Reader's Digest Condensed Books*, the first literature I ever owned. I peered out the window at the neighbours' home and the farm in the distance. I had recklessly climbed the ladders in the barn and jumped into the haylofts and learned how to milk a cow with the farmer's guidance. This was my first real home, where I felt secure. I would miss this familiar space.

Will I be homesick?

Mom and I shopped for a stylish new outfit for me to wear on my first day at the nurses' residence. I picked out a dark-patterned, long-sleeved sheath dress with a wide belted waistline and a V-neck. This was high fashion. The dress was simple and sophisticated, my choice guided by the teen magazines I regularly devoured.

I completed my outfit with black leather high-heeled shoes, and my swishy blonde hair had been trimmed to rest just above the collar. I thought I looked mature and ready for adventure.

I had always been well-dressed and advised all my female friends to "dress like a millionaire, because you never know who you might meet." I had a matching blue and cream leather luggage set. The smaller case was designed for an overnight stay and held toiletries—the soaps, shampoos, hair rollers, and a very small amount of makeup, as I didn't use more than pink blush and lipstick.

One suitcase in each hand, a small clutch purse under my arm, and I was ready to start the day that would change my life forever. My heart raced. I felt excited and nervous at the same time as I walked down the stairs to my waiting parents. I felt my shaking knees turn to jelly.

Leaving home for the first time left emotional tracks across my brain. *Will I ever move back to my bedroom? Is my childhood really finished? Do I truly want to be a nurse?*

The sun shone on my departure. How could I feel sad when I looked at my neighbours' old barn bathed in light, the stubble of the farm field soaking up the promise of next spring's growth?

"I'm ready to go." And so, it began.

Chapter 2

THE FIRST ORDER OF BUSINESS WAS A TEA TO BE held in the residence, a staid four-storey brick building set off to the side of the General Hospital. Renforth was a short drive from Saint John. Both Mom and Dad accompanied me, and we drove up the long hill of Waterloo Street to my new home. I was happy with their support and the effort they made to be with me. Dad found a parking spot and we all climbed out of the car, carrying my suitcases. I could hear the racket from outside the building.

What's all the noise? Sounds like a big party.

We walked up the front stairs to the entrance hall where I registered as a student. I was about to embark on a new path for my life. Excitement, sweat, anxiety, and a pounding heart underlay my calm outer demeanour. Was I thinking about nursing at that moment? No, I was hoping my new dress didn't have perspiration stains showing.

I was assigned room 417 in the centre wing of the

old residence. As my parents were about to get on the elevator, we were told men were not allowed to visit the floors. Dad was surprised but backed off the elevator.

I looked at him. "You okay with that?" I asked. As if he had a choice!

Rule number one had been pronounced, the first of many rules to come. Mom and I made our way to the small room with its metal bed. The room felt monastic. I placed some remnants of my childhood on the bed, including a few stuffed toys. The best part of the space was a large walk-in closet. The closet would become the after-bedtime study space where friends and I would cram for exams by the light of a lamp attached to a long extension cord—a definite no-no.

The thin mattress was covered with a striped spread, and pull drapes extended across a dirty window overlooking the rear parking lot. No apple trees or farmland in sight. The minimal decor included a study desk, chair, and very bare walls. A typed sheet, prominently placed on the desk, advised another rule, that the walls were not to be festooned with pictures.

The communal loo, with its toilet stalls and a few bathtubs to serve the entire wing of students, was near my room. The fourth floor contained a vintage, French-style metal cage elevator. It had a decorative bronze door that folded like an accordion and locked. It bumped its way up and down between floors, and the brick walls of the shaft were visible. Whenever I have a bad dream about a falling elevator, it is the vintage cage I recall.

I didn't immediately unpack. Mom and I made our way back down by the stairs to rejoin Dad. We took a brief look around the sitting rooms where we saw another rule posted in large print, underlined and bold: **Never shut the doors when entertaining a male friend.**

One small room had heart-shaped pillows, the only encouragement to the idea of romance. As people were coming and going all the time, what did they think students would get away with here? I had the feeling my dad liked this sign.

We entered the gymnasium where tables of sweets and pots of tea were set up to be shared by all of us as we chatted and introduced ourselves. I knew Jane Alexander, Donna Dobbin, and Janet Saunders from my high school class and saw familiar faces from other schools, who would soon become friends. The voices of seventy-six girls, their families, staff, and servers bounced off the walls in a cacophony of excited laughter, nervous giggles, twittery and shrieking voices, all of us simultaneously thinking about the looming departure time of family and the fact that we would soon be on our own.

"Mom? Dad? You don't have to stay to the very end. If you want to leave a bit sooner, I'm okay, go ahead." That was a lie. I wasn't okay, but I would never let on to that sinking feeling in my gut.

We were a room full of hopefuls about to embark on a nursing career. Most of us would make it.

Each probationer was assigned a mentor from the second-year students. They were there to help if the adjustment got rough and to share their own experiences with the challenges of the career. We wouldn't see each other very much, but the idea was comforting. My mentor, Pat Leach, was someone I'd known in high school, although we didn't share the same social circle. Pat had left me a note on top of the bedcovers explaining she would drop by after her evening shift ended.

I waited for her tap on the door. She entered my room, transformed from a high school beauty of the previous year into a sleek professional woman. She didn't stay long, but her visit reassured me. Somebody was looking out for me.

Will I look like her in a year? Can I change that much? Could I hope to emulate her wonderful, professional appearance? Could twelve months of training make such a difference in me?

I settled into the routine. Finding my way to class-rooms and the cafeteria was my first achievement. My first week was busy enough as I went to sick bay and labs to receive a series of injections designed to give protection from the variety of diseases I would ultimately come across. The worst of the lot was the live tuberculin bacillus, Bacillus Calmette-Guerin (BCG), scraped onto a patch of skin on the lower back over the spine. This was a brief procedure, resulting in an itchy scab and a slow healing process. I didn't want to be scratched with live bacteria, but given no choice, I obeyed the directive. Classmates coming out of the room looked distressed.

Tuberculosis had not been fully eliminated, and a full century before, a dedicated building behind the old hospital housed a sanatorium for those infected with the disease. Patients coughed up blood, alone in their misery and isolated from their families. Nurses and doctors were tasked with their care, at great risk to themselves. The nurses spent most of their time in the ward and thus had the greatest exposure. I marvelled at their courage in dealing with these cases, knowing full well their own personal risks.

Photographs taken seventy years earlier lined the hallways leading to our classrooms. Small numbers of young women—their long hair demurely held up in a bun, their caps perched on top of their heads, their floor-length uniforms covered in long aprons—posed for formal photographs. Where had they come from? Did they have families nearby, and what shaped their decisions to become nurses? The photographer must have said more than hold still. Did he also command, "Look serious, look professional"? Not one smile showed at the corners of the young women's mouths, but there they were, photographed in a split moment of time, faces caught in an image, but their stories never told.

Watching television, which had arrived in Saint John a mere five or six years before, wasn't a big part of a student's life. I was fourteen when I was invited to a friend's house to see their new TV, the first I'd ever seen. The only station, CBC, used a black-and-white image of the head of an Indigenous person to determine the focus and contrast for their programs. Saturday and Sunday nights were spent loving the hockey broadcasts, *The Ed Sullivan Show*, *The Jackie Gleason Show*, and a host of others. The young man whose father had purchased the TV suddenly became the most popular kid in the school. Night after night, a steady stream of teens landed at his house to watch the screen. Because of the lack of new programs in the early days of development, old Hollywood movies were rerun, and there were limited amounts of broadcast time.

The nurses' residence was limited to one television in the common room. The star attraction was baseball, not hockey. After work, when we could squeeze viewing time in, we gathered to cheer our own team on to victory. The room was dark, crowded, and stuffy. Heads got in the way, and senior students had the best choice of seats. There was no such thing as an individual television in a student's room, and Saturday night programs were replaced by late afternoon baseball. It didn't take me long to lose interest in this. In the same manner, my hours of lifeguarding and swimming at the YMCA pool in Saint John were now given up. I had enjoyed my athleticism as a teenager. Swimming, basketball, track and field, climbing, tennis, all of this came to a halt in the heavy commitment of hours and labour needed to become a competent nurse. I missed it, but those times were gone and fading fast from memory. I would have to find other ways to have moments of adventure.

Nursing students in 1959 studied from a modernized curriculum, in which many of us took our classes together in a block. Lecture time was taken out of our hours on duty. Ours was the largest class ever to be admitted, so inevitably we weren't all accommodated in the same room at once. While we were taught in the classroom and lab, we practiced short periods of time on the hospital wards under the supervision of the teaching staff or a head nurse.

Prior to our entrance in 1959, students had to make up classroom time, squeeze in study time, and get the required long hours of work experience on the ward. Work hours were exhausting, and students had only one half day off a week. A century earlier, time off was one half day and one Sunday a month. By 1959, attitudes were changing, and we were given one and a half days off a week. As probationers we were allowed to be absent on weekends. Those times were very special, and I don't believe we appreciated them until we lost them once we had regular nursing schedules and duties. The twenty-four-hour hospital day was broken into three eight-hour segments, and the shifts covered seven to three, three to eleven, and eleven to seven.

Our first orientation to the layout of the hospital gave us an overview of the wards and support services. Heads turned as we made our orderly way through the corridors, fresh-faced, ready for our chosen career, and walking like a gaggle of geese. I felt proud of my blue-striped uniform and gawked like a tourist. Visitors looked at us with curiosity.

I like this! I feel like somebody!

The residence was linked to the hospital by an underground tunnel, to be used in inclement weather. It gave me the creeps. Alone in it for the first time, I looked over my shoulder.

"Hello? Is anyone there?" Nobody answered. I had watched Alfred Hitchcock movies, in particular *Psycho*, and my overactive imagination triggered anxiety. It felt tomb-like underground. A thin sheen of moisture bathed the walls on rainy days. The air had a weird stale smell. I had wheels for feet as I picked up my pace and clutched my scissors in my hand.

The older section of the General Hospital had solariums at either end of the corridor. This had been forward-thinking so that patients who were ambulatory could sit in the sunroom and at least look out on a nice day. They could escape the smells of antiseptic, astringent, cleaners, and human waste and get away from the sounds of the hospital room.

Initially our classes took place in the lab in the classroom wing. We had mannequins to practice on and to learn the techniques that prepared us for the real thing, and we did the best job we could, pretending that in our care was a live human being. Of course, the only way to progress was to get to the wards as quickly as we could and begin the learning curve on something more than a stuffed rubber doll.

"You just killed your patient!"

The accusation might as well have been a slap in the face. My cheeks turned red in a wave of heat and denial, but the truth was obvious; my patient was on the floor by her bed.

"It was an accident! I didn't mean to!"

I looked at my patient, her neck bent backwards and one leg twisted under her knee. The nurse instructor glared furiously at me.

"Thank God she's a rubber dummy," I said.

Wrong choice of words. *Could I be expelled for this?*

"Pick her up, put her back together, and remember if she were human, you'd be on your way to jail."

I wiped the smirk off my face.

The lifelike mannequin was named Mrs. Chase. She smelled musty after years of being washed, dried, pierced, and probed during students' attempts to learn new skills. Often, she would land on the floor as we made her bed or gave her a bedpan or an injection.

Sorry, Mrs. Chase, I just dropped you on your head! Sorry, Mrs. Chase, the pan is stuck to your bottom.

The lab also housed a skeleton named Charlie. At some point in the distant past, he had been donated to medical science. We learned the names of all his bony parts. There are a lot of bones to know, and I hummed the Delta Rhythm Boys' version of "Dry Bones" as an aid to my memory.

"The thigh bone's connected to the hip bone; the hip bone's connected to the . . ." The song went around and around in my head.

Who were you? I wondered about this as I memorized Charlie's bony rack.

We learned how to do a proper bed bath, how to roll the patient across the bedding to change sheets, how to inspect the skin for pressure points and infection, and how to position a person on their side. The under sheet on the bed had to be rolled lengthwise while the draw sheet was held by another student on the opposite side of the bed. This was a time before fitted sheets and disposable moisture pads, so all linen had to be placed, pulled, and tightened without lumps or wrinkles that would disturb the skin. Then the entire procedure would be reversed. The top sheet had to be tucked in just so, in a toe-pressing right angle to the mattress. Over this was placed a cotton cover and a bedspread. We could fold the base of the sheet to loosen the pressure on toes, but rigorous attention was paid to the perfection and symmetry of the properly made bed. No patient could expose their feet. No one could tell me why that was.

I prepared for the real thing. What would a live patient be like? Reality would be a far cry from a mannequin. As probationary students, nursing without a bib covering the top of our blue pinstriped dresses gave a signal to the doctors, who knew immediately how much experience a student had. It was a great visual system.

Finally, the time came for me to experience a small amount of time on the ward, actually nursing a real person and not just the rubber dummy. My anxiety spiked, my armpits dampened, and my hands turned to ice. I tried not to show this as we practiced our limited knowledge for short periods on the wards, under close supervision.

From my diary, January 6, 1960

Today we mixed wards with classes, and I found it quite difficult. My anatomy notes are gone as well as my surgical scissors. I don't know where they went . . . or who took them, but suspect a certain classmate who never writes anything down!

This meant that I would have to borrow someone's notes and copy them into a fresh notebook so I could study in detail.

—ᴧᴧ—

We were learning something new every day, both in class and on the ward. Our first month of training, with its weekends off, came to a quick end. In the limited periods of time with patients, finally working with real people and not Mrs. Chase, we learned how to put our skills to use.

Despite living close to home, I experienced

homesickness, at times feeling sad and wishing for the easy and immature world of an eighteen-year-old. I wanted to sleep in my own bed and smell the delicious breakfast being cooked by my mom. I wanted to be free of the regimentation of the hospital. It was these times of sadness that I vented self-doubt into my pillow. How the students who had come from farther away managed to cope, I don't know. However, we were a sisterhood of nursing students forming the bonds that would hold us together through future decades.

As I look back to my nursing school friends, I marvel that I have continued my friendships with Donna and Janet, both of whom I met in grade three at Rothesay Consolidated School. Other classmates are also still part of my life—Pat Pettifer, Sue Weaver—and we periodically chat on the phone and share our lives' precious moments. If we still had a big closet to sit in, we would! I receive an annual class mailing list from Pat, and I share events in my life in a Christmas letter or an email to some of the remaining thirty-eight classmates.

Visual order was part of the basis for all order. The length of the sheet had to match on both sides of the bed, and the rubber drop sheet, covered in a linen cloth, had to be pulled so tight that a quarter dropped on its surface would bounce. I wondered about all these rules and who had devised them, and particularly, how far back in nursing history they had been initiated.

One head nurse was known to order that the entire bed be remade if the requisite bounce didn't happen when she tested the tightness of the drop sheet. She would tell one student to gather her classmates together in a designated patient's room.

"Make up the bed, Miss McCarthy."

I knew what was coming as I pulled the draw sheet with all my strength to get every fold out. A wrinkled sheet could imprint into the buttocks and result in a breakdown of the skin. All the students' eyes watched me as I made the effort to get it right.

The head nurse probably knew, well before she dropped the coin on the sheet, just how it would turn out. If the coin bounced, the sheet was perfect. The coin didn't bounce.

"Make it again and do it right."

Inevitably, if a patient peed the bed or worse, soiled it, the deposit did not always stay on the aptly named drop sheet. The entire bed would be stripped after the patient was washed. It didn't take us long to realize that patients moved about the bed, sunk lower down in it, and a lot of time would be spent cleaning up messes. My silent prayer was "Keep your bum in the middle." There were patients who I could swear peed the bed for attention. *Oh my God, she's gone again. Make her wait awhile.* That couldn't happen, of course, and the chronic piddlers resulted in two students helping each other and sharing the frequent task.

We would soon learn that bed making and mess cleaning fell predominantly on our shoulders, while the more important nursing tasks fell to the more experienced nurses.

Shockingly, we were not allowed to wear rubber gloves to protect ourselves from feces, and the job of cleaning a soiled bottom was an assault on the nose and hands. The odour would make me gag, and I would hold my breath until I turned a deep scarlet.

As I matured in nursing, I would often try to sneak a pair of surgical gloves to wear. There were no disposable gloves, and each pair was washed, tested for air tightness to indicate if the rubber was punctured, then autoclaved (steam sterilized) and wrapped up with the size marked on the package. Gloves were counted and reused, and a small supply was ordered for the doctors' use and for changing dressings. To be caught with a pair of gloves would go "on your record." Sneaking gloves could cause a shortage for a more strategic job than washing off poop. Bare hands or not, someone had to wash the patient's mess, and it was us.

Chapter 3

WHEN I HAD TIME, I CONTINUED TO DATE MY high school boyfriend. We would borrow a car, head to the movies, and drive over to the Reversing Falls Bridge to kiss and hug. Sometimes the city police would come along, shine a light in the car, and tell us to move on. It was good motivation not to go too far for fear of being arrested.

Everybody was changing and growing up as they headed off for college, military training, or entered demanding trades. They too had choices ahead and would follow new paths with people they met along the way. Our cohesive, chummy world was transforming right under our noses and would never regain its innocence. My special friend was on his way to another city to study engineering. It would be the end of our romance, the price we all paid.

At last, the day came when we were assigned full-time hours on the female surgery ward. It was our first eight-hour shift with real patients. We were finally leaving behind the musty rubber mannequin of the classroom for good and entering the hospital as a student nurse, ready to conquer the world.

On the way up to the ward I glanced at my friends. "Are you ready for this? Are you scared?" We all looked at one another, expectant but with sweaty hands and racing hearts. Our faces said it all.

Female surgery smelled of floor wax and urine. The equipment wasn't up to date. There were four heavy metal beds to a room, not one was electric, and I grunted as I manually cranked the handle attached to the frame to reposition the mattress. If the patient was heavy, the job took extra effort. The side rails manually slid up or down. The real aggravation was the set of four wheels, lined up perfectly, facing inward to one another, and in a straight line with the next bed. In the larger wards, the position of the wheels became more obvious. It is hard to describe the attitude of the head nurse, chastising us about this.

"Miss McCarthy, your wheels are not lined up. Go back in the room and do it over."

Crap. The toes of my black leather shoes were scuffed repeatedly when I kicked the rubber-coated wheels into submission. *Who the hell made these rules?*

There were no privacy screens attached to the ceiling. Portable metal screens with white cotton covers were moved back and forth when needed.

The tiny gap at each edge didn't ensure privacy. When the screens were not in use, they were folded up and placed against the wall.

After a patient used the bedpan, I placed a plain cotton cover over the contents and walked it down the hall to the "dirty" utility room. It was my job to clean the pan then return it to the bedside cupboard. As I walked by with the soiled contents, visitors would give me a pitying look. At those times I thought, *And why did I choose this profession?*

When a patient was discharged, the cleaning of the bed and all the equipment was the responsibility of the student. We stripped and washed every inch of the frame and mattress cover with boiling hot, soapy water. We carried the dirty bedding down the hall to the laundry chute and tossed it in. It whooshed down the tube, sending back a blast of smelly air into our faces. We made up the bed with fresh linens and stocked the bedside table. Infection control was a big part of what we did, although we didn't recognize the fact. I don't recall a ward ever having infectious outbreaks, and it is to the meticulous cleaning routines carried out by students that the credit goes.

In the classroom, we were introduced to the mystery of tubes. I learned the use for a rectal tube: to put soap suds and liquid in the bowel so that it could empty itself or to allow gas out.

The role-playing on Mrs. Chase didn't prepare me for the experience of giving an enema to a real person. Working on female surgery, I received the nursing report and had my orders for my shift. Included in the lengthy list were enemas, dressing changes, blood pressure monitoring, temperature and pulse recordings, bed baths, and one lice treatment.

I kept a notebook in my pocket and, during report, wrote the details of my patient's requirements with as much speed as I could. Each task completed was later recorded on their chart. In addition, I made rounds with doctors, took patients to X-ray, and dealt with all manner of other interruptions to my work.

I was about to give an enema and pretended I wasn't shy and inexperienced. I felt embarrassed and horrified at the thought of poking a tube in a patient's behind. I cleaned the anal area with soap and water, soaking her enough to clean the backside of a cow. I watched the water dribble onto the bedding and knew I would have to change all the linen. I lubricated the rectal tube, hung the suds enema bag on a pole by the bed, clamped off the tube, and stood back to decide how far to insert it. I crossed my fingers, thinking, *I hope it doesn't land in her stomach.*

"Mrs. Smith, I'm going to give you an enema. I want you to roll on your side, so I can put the tube up your bum." This sounded unprofessional, but

I had to judge whether or not to use anatomical words. "Take a deep breath, while I put the tube in."

I followed my own instructions and sucked in a great breath of air, then spread her buttocks and inserted the tube. And waited.

Nothing happened. Absolutely nothing.

Then, I remembered to unclamp the tube so the suds could flow. And flow they did. The quick rush of soapy water entering her rectum should have been accompanied by my instruction to her, "Hold it, hold it. Tighten, don't let it go," or something to that effect. But I was still holding my own breath and hoping that she didn't release the whole mess of soap, water, and poop onto the bed.

Mrs. Smith yelled, "I've got to shit!"

Lordy, how exact those words were. I pushed her out of the bed.

"Hurry up! Get in the bathroom!"

Quick, quick, but not quick enough. Clutching her Johnny shirt to her backside, she dribbled a few bits on the floor and hit the toilet on the run. She produced explosive sounds that reverberated around the ward, given that I had forgotten to shut the door.

I left her and dashed from the room in search of a mop and bucket and ran right into a handsome doctor. He was my mother's general practitioner, and I grabbed his arm, in one of life's embarrassing moments. I clutched him and hugged him.

"Dr. Freedman, I just gave my first enema! I'm so excited!"

He looked at me with an expression that said, "Not only are you blonde, but you're also a dumb blonde."

Mopping the floor brought me back to reality.

My learning curve continued on female surgery. I was about to catheterize a lady, and I wasn't ready for the experience. How easy it had been on Mrs. Chase, with her large, hairless, clearly seen openings.

This patient was unable to pee after surgery. Too many hours had ticked by. Intervention with a catheter was essential. I fetched the treatment tray along with two additional tubes just in case. I explained to her what I intended to do, failing to mention that this was my first time.

"Ma'am, have you gone to the bathroom in the last several hours?" I hoped she would answer yes, so I could get out of doing this task, but her answer was a definitive no.

My mind was my cheerleader.

You can do this, Francene.

No, I can't.

Yes, you can.

My patient was obese. And very hairy. I knew she had birthed three children a few years apart, and that she was well managed for pain. I sat her on a bed pan, hoping she could go. Alas, no luck, so I washed her perineum with soapy water.

We'd been drilled about cleanliness and a sterile field. An oxymoron, in this case, if there ever was one. Her belly hung down over her pubic bone, and I had to position a lamp between her legs, to get a better view.

My gosh, she's fat everywhere. What a shameful thought.

"Now, ma'am, this may sting a bit." Pulling surgical gloves on, I positioned the sterile bowl to catch the pee once it started to flow.

I looked for the urethral opening. I looked some more. Nowhere could I see what I had easily observed in the student lab. Mrs. Chase had such a clear plastic urethra. The overhanging belly fat, and more fat, obliterated the location.

Ah! Got it! Or so I thought.

"There you go, dear, take a nice deep breath, I'm just going to insert the catheter and it might sting a bit." Insert I did, but the tube folded back on itself as I realized I had poked it into a fold of fat.

"I'm sorry, ma'am. I'm going to try again."

Round two and no urine flowed. This time I had aimed it into her vagina. I blushed, apologized, and asked, "Did I hurt you?"

She roared with laughter and replied, "I've had bigger things in there, let alone three babies that came out."

The other patients in the room shrieked with laughter, and I wished the floor would open up and swallow me whole. I headed out to the utility room for a fresh catheter and gloves. I returned to a strangely quiet room where I observed the foreboding glare of the head nurse.

She hovered by my patient, no doubt attracted by the raucous laughter.

"Are you experiencing difficulties, Miss McCarthy?" she asked.

"No, I just contaminated the catheter."

The head nurse left in a swish of starch. I proceeded to reassess the location of the urethra, aided by a four-by-four-inch square of gauze to move the abundant flesh aside. Then I had a brilliant idea.

"Could you pull your belly up with both hands?" I asked.

That did it. I found the right spot. The urine flowed abundantly and filled the bowl to the top.

Another successful moment in the life of a student, except for one thing. I had forgotten to have an instructor observe me. A record was kept of each treatment I did until I was deemed skilled enough not to require supervision.

Female surgery always had an interesting population of patients. Occasionally a prostitute would be admitted and treated for the disorders of the trade. My friend Donna remembers a prostitute telling her,

"My dear, I don't know why you work so hard when you're sitting on a million dollars!" I don't know how much money a prostitute managed to keep, but it had to be more than our Victorian-era six dollars a month.

I wrote in a diary in my first year, but beyond that time, I was too busy and didn't maintain it very often. We learned in the classroom and took further training by observing procedures on the wards, where doctors performed tests and procedures as we stood by, wide-eyed and shaking. There was one procedure that I did note.

From my diary, February 18, 1960

I watched an abdominal paracentesis and got sick! Ooh, I darn near fainted along with four other girls. The doctor drained a quart of fluid from the abdomen of a carcinoma patient and then sutured her. I felt so badly for the poor soul.

Except for visiting hours, hospitals were very quiet. No loud talk in the corridors at night, no joking and laughing out loud to disturb the patients. It was a serene and hallowed atmosphere.

There was no such thing as a hospital television,

radios were not allowed, and staff went quietly about their duty. The noisiest room was the "dirty" utility area where the clank of pans and equipment could be heard along with the gurgle of flushes and running taps. At visiting hour, the ambient noise picked up as all the visitors descended on the wards around the same time. Patients in pain broke the quiet, yet overall, the atmosphere was a study in managed calm. The noises of retching, coughing, gasping, farting, belching, snoring, and all the elements of the human condition were easily heard. Our ears were trained to listen to the sounds of the person, not just the bell buzzing over the room door.

Diabetic urine testing was a chore. At regular intervals I would go through my list of patients and their required treatments to ascertain from whom urine had to be collected to monitor the presence of sugar. As the level built up in the bloodstream, it spilled over into the urine, and careful testing established what amount of insulin would be injected. There were no handy digital machines, no quick prick with a lancet to the finger. I gathered a bedpan or urinal and asked the patient to provide a sample. Some did, some didn't, and some had just peed in the toilet. Depending on that, the entire timing of medicating with insulin could be thrown off. After a successful piddle, I poured the contents of the pan into a pitcher, then took it to the utility room.

This pee reeks. I couldn't pinch my nose at the same time as I held droppers and tubes.

Testing was a smelly process, as diabetic urine had a sickly-sweet smell indicating the presence of sugar. The importance of this couldn't be underestimated, as insulin injections were adjusted according to the level of sugar present. Using a glass dropper to suck up the urine, I carefully counted so many drops into the test tube and then dropped in a tablet that fizzled and turned into a readable colour after one minute. I matched the now pigmented pee sample to a cardboard monitoring strip and obtained the reading, which I wrote down in my notebook to be transferred right away to a graph sheet on the patient's chart. Once all that was done, the dropper and tube had to be cleaned and placed back in the rack. The effects of sugar spilling into the bloodstream and kidneys had significant impacts on the body's major organs, the circulatory blood vessels, the eyes, and the neuropathic nerve endings of the vascular bed. Diabetes was part of my own family history, so I took this task very seriously.

Friday was always fish day, and the aroma wafted all through the hospital. The kitchen aides plunked the food tray down on the bedside table with no effort to see if the patient could reach it, let alone if they were awake. I dashed from room to room, making sure no one had been missed, hand cranked up beds, rolled tray tables into place, and helped patients with their meals. Patients who were infirm and frail were fed, and because there were never enough hands to go around, the food had to be popped into the patient's mouth quickly. Often the kitchen staff were back to pick up the trays before people had even gotten started.

Feeding someone, I am ashamed to admit, was a job I hated. Soup would dribble down chins, chewed bits hung off the lip, and drool came down from the corners of the mouth—all in all not what I expected nursing to be. But then, what did I know about the real world of the elderly and infirm and the decline of bodily function? After breaking all speed-feeding records, I needed to tidy faces and hands, and sometimes a fresh Johnny shirt was in order. On the evening shift, I took around stacks of toast and jam, juice or water, and gave out the bedtime snacks. There would come a time when this would be done by paid helpers.

We studied pharmacology, learning an encyclopedic amount about drugs, painkillers, mood-altering psychotropics, antibiotics, anti-inflammatories, hypnotics, correct dosing, allergic reactions, and how to set up a drug tray. If you were assigned drug duty, all the prescription cards were cross-referenced to the doctor's orders in the chart and to the tracking system called a cardex.

I assembled the pill bottles and a metal tray holding paper pill cups. The individual patient card was inserted into a clip by the cup then carefully read and compared with the supply bottle of the prescription, and only then did the drug get placed in the cup. I learned the meaning of acronyms like qod (once a day), q4h (every four hours), tid (three times a day), and so on. Drug rounds had to be at the prescribed times.

At each patient's bedside, the card was read, compared to the patient's name band, and the pill handed over to be taken immediately. There was no walking away and leaving it for later. It had to be consumed at once in the presence of the nurse. The words no drug nurse ever wanted to hear were "That's not my pill!" Or "Is that a new pill?" Or "It's not the same colour as the last one!" Mistakes were not tolerated, yet they did happen at times. I feared making a mistake. I'm not sure if that fear was for my fate or that of the patient.

Painkilling drugs were carefully dispensed from a locked cupboard, the key to which was always in the control of the head nurse. Narcotic medication could only be dispensed with two nurses present to witness and monitor it: the head nurse with the key and the student tasked with its administration. Not all products were in ready-to-use form. Some narcotics were pills that had to be dissolved for use.

Anytime I see a tiny teaspoon I recall the nursing procedure. Sterile water was heated in a teaspoon over the flame of a Bunsen burner. The tiny pill was dropped on this, dissolved, then sucked up into the syringe for injection, either subcutaneously in the skin of the upper arm or as an intramuscular into the gluteus maximus muscle of the buttocks with a much larger needle.

"Roll over, sir, I have a little needle to give you. It won't hurt a bit." The needle was almost two inches in length, and if the skin was thin, the response from the patient was an audible "Ouch!"

Some narcotics were contained in glass ampules. The glass neck had to be snapped off to get at the liquid within, and the supervising nurse stood by to inspect the procedure. If by chance during the snapping of the neck the glass broke and contaminated the contents, it was dumped and flushed down the sink then signed off by two nurses as "wasted." Begin again.

At the end of the shift, the nurse in charge, along with the student who did the drug count, cross-checked that what was in the locked cupboard matched the records of use, then signed the control book. The oncoming nurse in charge went through the count again with the previous holder of the keys.

The only weak link in this system was the lack of control over sleeping pills. No record of use was maintained. Large bottles filled with red Seconal tablets or yellow-and-black Nembutal were in the cupboard. It was inevitable that times of sleep deprivation occurred from working on night shift. Sometimes when we were the student dispensing meds and were asked to unlock the cupboard, we would help ourselves to a sleeping pill to take later when sleep would not come naturally.

"What do you have more of, the Seconal or the Nembutal?" We wouldn't dare ask the nurse in charge but only chance the request with a fellow student.

A glance would show which was in greater supply, and it would be from the fuller bottle that the capsule would come. It didn't take very long for the dispensing pharmacists to recognize that pills were being nipped, and the practice was put in place to record these hypnotic drugs in the same manner as narcotics. The abuse was not widespread, and as students we had the option to go to sick bay, explain the problem, and perhaps then be given a sleeping pill for one use only.

Pain control was not a well-established process; monitored intravenous drug therapy was decades into the future. Many patients suffered needless excruciating pain while they waited for the requisite time between doses to elapse. There was no way a narcotic drug could be administered earlier than ordered, no matter the dire straits of the patient.

One male patient would stay in my memory forever. Elderly, dying from bowel cancer, skin and bones holding his six-foot frame together, he was eaten by pain that broke his spirit and drained his courage. He was only allowed 100 mg of Demerol every four hours. His pain broke through every two hours, and his groans turned to screams coming from inside his soul with every breath. The last hour before his medicine could be given, he would cry out repeatedly at the top of his lungs until exhaustion knocked him back for a few minutes. Then he began again. His sounds were feral and unrelieved, and we would try to assuage him by the simplest and ineffective measures of rubbing his arms or washing his back, to no avail.

A few times I drew up his Demerol ahead of schedule only to be told, "No, you can't give it early." What was the sense of worrying about addiction in a dying man? The doctors didn't have to listen to his ferocious cries making his throat raw, but the other patients in the ward did, and the nurses. I finally spoke with his doctor when he came in for rounds.

"He needs more Demerol, sir. He screams

constantly and no human being should have to go through that."

My tears welled up, as I was assigned to this suffering man, and it was more than I could personally deal with. His situation created such empathy in me that I would go off duty still hearing him. The doctor listened to me, and that gave me a great feeling of relief.

I'm not sure what the outcome would have been had the head nurse heard my intervention. In any event, the patient's pain management was somewhat modified, and despite it being more than a half century later as I write this, I recall his name and I see him yet, in his extremis.

One of the more archaic nursing practices was the making of a poultice. In centuries past, before the advent of antibiotics, lung congestion could rapidly lead to death. The remedy was to make a hot poultice. It worked as well in 1959 as it did through the ages.

Sometimes the poultice was a pan of fried onions, their pungent aroma enough to water the eyes and clear the nose. I cooked the ingredients on the stove then wrapped the mixture in cheesecloth followed by an outer towel for placement on the patient's chest. The hot bundle increased circulation and helped draw out infection. Linseed was another product of choice, boiled to a congealed, porridge-like consistency, dumped into cheesecloth, covered in flannel, and applied. The intense heat left a large warm pink ring on the skin. This broke up thick mucus. Practices that sound strange now had a sound basis in science and were effective. Mustard plaster applications worked in the same way.

I learned how to change a dressing over an infected incision oozing pus. Suture material would break down and leave gaping holes. A dirty, debris-filled wound festered, and the task of cleaning and re-dressing it fell to the student.

The "clean" utility room housed sterilized and wrapped dressing trays. I would carefully open the tray and pour saline water in one stainless bowl and green antiseptic soap in the other. Undressing the bandage and removing adhesive tape was accompanied by groans as it was peeled away then discarded. The antiseptic soap was used to clean off dried or wet secretions using Kelly forceps (a versatile instrument used to clamp blood vessels in an operation, but also commonly used to hold the gauze squares when doing a dressing) and gauze squares, before rinsing with saline water. Then fresh gauze was placed over the skin and snugly held in place with adhesive tape. Sometimes an antibiotic in powder form was applied as an extra precaution.

I never knew what to expect when undoing a dressing. The presence of a foul smell was the first indication of infection. Some wounds actually frothed, and with the patient enclosed in a small room behind a screen, the air grew putrid and induced my gag reflex. I clearly recall those unpleasant moments. One woman's stitches had become infected overnight, and the entire abdominal area was soaked and floating in pus. As I removed the gauze, several layers of her skin peeled away, and I grabbed the bed screen by its edge to keep from fainting.

"Oops. I dropped my pen, just a sec." A very long sec! Who was I fooling? No nurse worth her salt would faint, and I leaned over, pretending to look for my pen while the blood returned to my head. Being lightheaded and the dizzy near miss of fainting left me with a sweat-beaded face, but I finished the job, wrapped up all the debris, and left the room as fast as my wobbly legs could carry me away. I had to ask permission to return to the nurses' residence to change my uniform to get rid of the cloying smell of rotting flesh clinging to my clothes.

How will I ever complete my training? That thought tormented me. I didn't believe I had the right amount of toughness to stay the course. The first year had only just gotten underway, and my self-doubt was building. Occasionally this was shared with my mentor or other students. We were all having challenges.

From my diary, January 30, 1960

Hell's bells! Today no class time and I absolutely detest it. I did a gruesome dressing on a woman's foot with gangrene. Half of it was rotted away.

Chapter 4

TIME WAS FLYING BY. I HAD LEARNED SO MUCH IN a few short months, and there was still a huge learning curve ahead. The long starched aprons were okay, and the military-style shoes were comfortable, even at the end of eight hours standing on my feet.

Black shoes required frequent polishing with cleaning cream. Old rags did the trick, and a brush buffed the leather. I had watched my father do a daily cleaning of his shoes, sitting them on old newspapers, so I knew the right way to get a military shine on my own footwear.

There was a fixed routine to our days. Up at 5:45 a.m., a quick wash in the loo, dressing in black stockings, shoes, blue-and-white pinstriped dress, collar attached, apron done up at the back, and scissors tucked into place. I would grab my wool cape and dash down the back stairs, followed by a run across the courtyard to the hospital waiting area where morning roll call was performed. It always felt rushed.

Name after name was read aloud, followed by a response.

"McCarthy." A very brief pause, then, "Present!"

The roll call was followed by a short Bible reading and the Lord's Prayer. This all took place at 6:30 a.m., leaving very few minutes to line up in the cafeteria, wolf down some breakfast (I loved a bowl of porridge smothered in brown sugar, with toast and tea), and then run up the back stairs to get on the ward by 7:00 a.m., in time to hear the night nurse's report.

While working on the ward, there was no chance to take a sit-down break except to do some brief manual charting. Our time for lunch was another short thirty minutes, squeezed into the day whenever we were told we could leave to eat. We scrambled to line up in the cafeteria, which reduced our eating time to somewhere under twenty minutes. This was followed by another dash up the stairs to the ward. There was no time to brush teeth or return to the residence unless you chose to skip your meal.

Needless to say, there were no computers back then. A wall of cubby spaces held each chart in place, and a large cardex, numbered room by room, held a corresponding note on each patient. The head nurse copied all doctors' daily orders into the system and noted pertinent facts about each person at every shift. Thus, changes in vital signs, noteworthy information, and meds were recorded and read in their entirety to the oncoming staff and students.

Even as probationers, we had life-and-death responsibilities on the wards, but in residence we were treated like children. We were governed by a staff of "white ladies"—not a reference to their race but rather to their white uniforms. They oversaw all coming and going of the students in residence, and we were required to be inside no later than 11:00 p.m., except for a few late-night passes a month, allowing us to return by 1:00 a.m., all diligently recorded and noted on our student card. Our room lights had to be extinguished by 11:15 p.m. The ladies, with their flashlights, made the rounds of every floor, shining their torches and listening at doors if they thought they heard anything out of the ordinary. If I was caught with my room lamp on, they walked right in and demanded it be turned off.

There I was, responsible for serious work with patients but not allowed to regulate my bedtime or my lights out. When extra study was needed for tests, students squeezed into each other's closets to cram and quiz. We rigged up an extension cord inside the closet and grabbed some extra study time or shared a whispered conversation we deemed important. It was hot and stuffy, but it worked. Many a friendship was forged in those moments of flouting the rules.

Finally, we took our first set of exams, a make-or-break experience that would see a few of us depart for other pastures. Writing our exams was intended to separate the "wannabe" nurses from those who would really set their sights on success. We all started out with that common goal, but sometimes it was just too much, and a few of our classmates left after the marks were posted. Our brains were stuffed full. We wrote, and most of us passed, the exams for anatomy and physiology, pharmacy, and medical and surgical nursing, to name a few. Our student body shrank from seventy-nine to sixty-one students after the first set of marks were posted.

Seventy-one hours of lecture time and nine hours of lab time in anatomy and physiology—including chemistry, my nemesis—resulted in a grade of 85 percent. Drug therapy took up forty-five hours of instruction, and I was up to speed on a vast number of medications, their side effects, proper dosing, allergic reactions, and age-appropriate and disease-appropriate medicine. I checked the doctors' medical orders and on very rare occasions was able to detect an error and bring it to the head nurse's attention. Twenty-six hours of lecture time were allocated to microbiology, along with fifteen hours of lab time. For that subject I received a mark of 80 percent.

However, a book can't replace practical learning. Thirty-four hours of lecture time and reading about human psychology could only touch on that vastly complex subject.

I had looked forward to being away from the General and doing a stint at the psychiatric hospital, having been a keen reader of *The Complete Psychological Works of Sigmund Freud*. Not ordinary reading for a young woman, to be sure, but the dynamics of the human mind fascinated me. Given the large number of students in our class, we could not all be assigned the same work experiences. There was no psych unit in the General. The other option was a week-long placement with the Victorian Order of Nurses, partnering with a registered nurse (RN) and tagging along on calls to patients in need of home care.

I also completed nineteen hours of diet therapy, some of which were spent in the vast kitchens servicing the hospital. I had no idea an entire butchered steer could hang so huge. The butchers and chefs on rare occasions would cut off a choice steak for a few of us, which I then had to smuggle from the kitchen, wrapped in brown paper and hidden beneath my wool cape.

I had visions of traipsing across the yard, dripping a red trail of blood behind me. The meat would then be pan-fried with onions in the residence kitchen, and the smell would waft out to the corridors.

"Steak's on, come and get it!" Delicious for anybody able to get a bite, and it was quickly consumed.

Being hungry a lot of the time seemed to accompany our level of hard work. I lived on ice cream floats in the cafeteria, peanut butter on crackers in the residence, and the sustaining offerings of Bruns Restaurant across Waterloo Street. Bruns's claim to fame rested on three sandwich offerings: chicken salad, ham salad, and egg salad. These were washed down with rich, delicious milkshakes. The Bruns family made their living feeding starving students. My nutrition studies produced a mark of 90 percent, attesting to my love of food, no doubt!

Chapter 5

PROBATIONERS NO LONGER! AFTER FIVE MONTHS of finding our way, dressed in a pinstriped dress and apron, we were awarded the coveted plain white cap and bib.

From my diary, January 25, 1960

Tonight was capping night and it started at eight o'clock officially. We got our bibs and then moved into the auditorium, where the guests were gathered. We got our caps, put them on, and received our white candles. Then the candlelight service began. We received white leather New Testament Bibles from the Gideon's International. I received, all together, twelve dollars from Mom and Dad and Sis. What a thrill!

The administration made us feel very special, holding a candlelight ceremony in the nurses' residence. It felt great to have the cap placed on my head while my proud parents looked on. *They must have come in early, to be seated in the third row. They're proud of me, I can see it in their faces, and oh, my stomach is fluttering! Butterflies! I can't believe I have a cap on my head after all my doubts. Mental hug, Francene. Stand tall!*

I winked at them.

The guest speaker was Margaret MacPhedran from the University of New Brunswick. She spoke of the qualities of courage and hard work. She was correct on the hard work aspect, and our courage would slowly build. Wearing that little piece of starched white handkerchief was a proud moment based on a very long history of nursing.

We would soon discover the downside to wearing the cap, knocking it against room screens and bed rails when leaning over to do our work. Bobby pins, lots of them, to the rescue.

The new sense of a sisterhood was tempered by the reality of the pecking order amongst first, second, and third-year students. We did not crowd into an elevator full of seniors. We often walked up the stairs. Unspoken and unwritten rules were absorbed by osmosis and example, and we were aware of an air of restraint. There was not much back and forth between the full student body, and our housing arrangements kept us separated. The doctors recognized that a new cap did not a nurse make, and it was to the senior students, with their white stockings and shoes to mark their rank, that they turned to when on the wards. Nevertheless, it was a good system because it worked.

From my diary, February 3, 1960

Thirteen girls (February class) graduated today, and they sang their grad songs about hospital life at breakfast—all about bedpans, perineal care, etc. What a wonderful feeling for them to be done.

(Note: This was the last class of graduates who had entered the nursing school at a time when there were two student intakes per year.)

My next duty roster took place on male surgery. My experience here was not much different from female surgery. The men bore their challenges with stoic dignity for the most part, and personal care was performed by male orderlies. The myth about nurses knowing so much about male anatomy was just that. The closest I came to a man's nether region was to hand over a urinal and come back later for it. Even that induced me to blush.

Male surgery was graced by Hallie. He was a paraplegic who spent his days in the hospital ward, becoming almost a fixture, a long-term patient with an indwelling catheter. He was so frustrated, confined to bed, watching the young student nurses every day, and likely fantasizing about a hot date. Once in a while, he would get overly excited and his eyes would spark, accompanied by his attempt to grab a quick touch, almost succeeding. We all warned him. "Hey! Settle down! Don't try that again!"

We grew used to his antics and were not insulted. Rather, we developed a sense of compassion for this middle-aged man robbed of the full use of his limbs. If we were irritated by him, he became the topic of jokes. Other times we pulled his screen around his bed, sensing his need for privacy.

In male surgery, tasks were similar to those in female surgery. I did bed baths, back rubs, dressings, urine testing, meds, and checked blood pressure and vital signs, just like any other part of the hospital.

The head nurse was Miss Gaunce. Her severe demeanour scared me. The common characteristic of all head nurses was their shared disdain for nursing students, while they maintained a look of immaculate, unwrinkled, and starched professionalism. I always wondered if the laundry put extra starch in their uniforms. A few hours into the duty period, all students were rumpled and a bit messed from the myriad duties they performed on top of their nursing work. Cleaning rumpled us.

If a student had any doubts at all about the pecking order of the hospital, they were magnified in the rarefied atmosphere at the nursing station. When the doctors came around, we all stood up to show our respect, no matter what aspect of charting or reviewing we were engaged in. Doctors were like God, held in awe and never questioned. They wrote illegibly, grabbed charts, looked at them, and then threw them on the desk, not caring if the papers dislodged. They left in a whirlwind to make the rounds of their patients. After each eminent presence departed, the chart was scanned for new orders, med changes were noted, requisitions were made out for new tests, and all the information was updated on the cardex system.

Soon I would be reporting for work from 3:00 p.m. to 11:00 p.m. Working the day shift from 7:00 a.m. to 3:00 p.m. was short-lived, as were weekends off. I was now regularly scheduled on evenings and nights, all too often. I quickly found out that my days off might be split up.

The impact on romance was enormous, as my special friend at university only had weekends off. There were split shifts, and on some Saturdays, I worked an hour or two in the afternoon, then went back to work hours later. It was a challenge to plan meaningful time together, and it began to strain our romance to the breaking point. Simply put, nursing came first.

The evening shift had a different rhythm than

days. I listened to the complete nursing report, made notes of room numbers and which patients had been assigned to me, then quickly checked the cardex to record the number of dressings, vitals, and urine tests. It was not unusual to be taking care of eight patients.

Even at this early stage of my student days, I got to see and experience death. I was never prepared for my emotional reaction. I had lost grandparents at an early age, but in the hospital setting of suffering and administering care, it resonated at a different level. I was working the evening shift when the following happened.

From my diary, March 1, 1960

At 3:30 p.m., on evening shift, a man died, and suddenly I realized what medicine was: the doctor listening to the patient's heart, the emergency oxygen, and the final stimulant injection. Then nothing. Just a shell, where once there was a live being with a soul.

Throughout the evening shift I thought a lot about his death. It had come quickly and quietly, without family present to hold his hand or say a few comforting words.

I have often thought about the power of touch. I learned early in my nursing career that respectful human touch conveyed a wealth of unspoken compassion and love. It was the silent language that reached through barriers of pain and fear.

To be simply present in another's space, to share a time of profound challenge, to make a connection with another person was all part of a nurse's role. I knew I possessed the gift of energy flowing through my hands and that it worked in a mysterious way that I couldn't understand.

The loving intention behind healthy touch crosses energetic barriers and bridges through the chaos of pain. To be suffering alone is a wretched experience. Accompanying the patient in their journey, being present to their need, is a shared bond of being human. Nurses know that. They all have their experiences.

At 4:00 p.m. during evening shifts, everyone's vitals had to be recorded: temperature, pulse, and respiration rate. Sometimes students were assigned this task for all the patients on the ward.

"McCarthy, you've got all the temperatures today."

I didn't dare roll my eyes at this pronouncement, but I thought it was unfair. After an hour of shaking down the thin thread of mercury contained in the glass thermometer, my wrist, elbow, and shoulder throbbed. It took so much time to do them all, and I would rush from room to room with the words "I'll be right back." Often, I wasn't. The patients took their own action after a long wait for my return.

"Oh, I'm sorry," I would say, as I found some thermometers hanging out of mouths, others put back in their stainless-steel container, and still others just lying on the bedding, in danger of being broken. All the results were noted on graph sheets in the chart and on the cardex.

Supper was delivered to the floors at five o'clock, and I helped those who needed assistance. This was followed by a mad dash to distribute toothbrushes and toothpaste to patients before their visitors arrived at seven.

I would rush into the room, saying in a cheery, singsong voice, "Time to get cleaned up," and wondering if the people took as much care at home.

—∿—

As was the case when I visited a patient with my mother when I was eight, in the 1960s hospitals had limited visiting hours. Hordes of family and friends would arrive in a flurry, jamming elevators and pushing down the halls to see their loved ones. Visiting was supposed to last an hour, although many folks tried to stretch the time out for an extra half hour.

All of this took place alongside dressings, meds, and tests for diabetics, while I answered patients' room buzzers. I carried loaded but covered bedpans down the hallway, which elicited sympathetic or disdainful glances. The looks said, "Who in their right mind would do this job?" I wondered about that myself at times.

The rate of room bell ringing peaked at 9:00 p.m. The over-the-door mounted lights would flash along with the buzzers. An impatient, often desperate patient would yell, "Nurse! Nurse! Nurse!" in a progressively demanding tone, no matter how fast I responded. Some people I thought were frail and feeble could bellow with the best of them!

Visitors made their own requests too, coming to the nursing station to ask questions about the meds, whether the doctor had been in, and in general relaying any concern the patient had. Sometimes they treated us as though we were ignorant, and if our answers weren't good enough, they would demand to see the head nurse, who might and usually did give the same response we had given.

Patience was always the prerequisite. Once visitors left and our assigned tasks were completed, we prepared the wash basins and cleaned hands, faces, backs, and any other body part. We also provided a thorough back rub. This was not just a nicety but gave an opportunity to check the condition of the skin on patients who were confined to bed. Bedsores or pressure spots could become seriously infected. No nurse worth her salt would ignore the skin care routine and the peril posed by a bedsore.

It was virtually unheard of that a pressure wound would occur, given the stringent observations we made and the care we gave. The proximity of the pressure point on the lower back to the spinal cord meant that an infection could travel quickly and be life-threatening.

Preparing patients for bedtime included oral care, which was not my favourite job. However, not liking it didn't make the task go away. The stainless-steel tooth container was kept discreetly in the bedside drawer until I removed it and filled it with water. I dropped the false teeth into it and little flecks of supper floated to the top. I resisted the urge to gag and charged into the bathroom. I would run a heavy stream of water, dump the contents, pick up the teeth, and brush them. Remember, we were not allowed to wear gloves. I no longer believed the dentifrice ads that said, "No brushing needed"!

Invariably my gag reflex kicked in and, superimposed over the sound of the running water, resulted in the sound of me coughing in a peculiar way inside the bathroom. The spotless teeth were returned to the bedside table, floating in water, and all would be well when a toothless, pucker-mouthed smile accompanied a thank you from the apple-doll face looking up from the bed. Those of us with a full set of teeth may not know how the toothless face looks.

Once all medical tasks were done, housekeeping

chores were squeezed in. Flower bouquets were refreshed, bedside paper bags were replaced, and the general untidiness of the ward and personal belongings were looked after. Nursing duties really were a complete package, performed by the student without any auxiliary help.

Just before the shift changed, I would sit at the nursing desk to record eight hours of information onto the chart and cardex. Once the night nurses were ready to take over and the report ended, many students would gather in the cafeteria for a late-night round of toast or ice cream floats. Then it was off to bed for well-earned sleep. Unless you were reporting for duty again at 7:00 a.m.

Chapter 6

NIGHT SHIFT! I DON'T THINK I KNEW WHAT A BIO-rhythm was back in my student days. I just knew that my body couldn't stand the task of keeping itself awake and alert all night, or the reverse in the morning when I needed to go to sleep and couldn't. I tried earplugs, eye masks, and evening naps, all to no avail.

The result was an exhausted student with a per-petual sleep deficit. I never had enough hours of restorative sleep, and this was exacerbated by the busy, noisy residence. My room was near the com-munal loo, and I heard every toilet flushed, every bath drawn, every sink used, clicking heels on the tile floor, giggling gossip, radios, ambulance sirens— all manner of racket.

On my first night duty, I had to check the blood pressure of a very ill patient whose vitals were unsta-ble. Every fifteen minutes, for several hours, I walked in and pumped up the cuff on his arm. By morning

I was seeing it inscribed in my brain. When I finally fell asleep, I awoke exactly every fifteen minutes.

On duty, I struggled to keep myself awake and alert. The start of the shift was the busiest time; however, every patient's room had to be visited hourly throughout the night.

Why the hell am I going into a room with a flashlight, just after getting him to settle? This is crazy!

It appeared as though I was purposely creating a sleep deficit in the patients, but this practice was a requirement. Sometimes the rules were a mystery. Why we did this so often eluded me, as invariably, popping in and out carrying a flashlight and playing its beam onto the bed would disturb any light sleeper. Walking up the long dark corridor, flashlight in hand, gave me the jitters.

Oh my God. What is that sound? That can't be human. Yes, it is, and it sure isn't snoring.

The hallways were almost pitch-dark. The lack of light created shadows and fuelled my anxiety. At the far end of the corridor, I could hear the rattling sound of a congestion-filled chest. The man was struggling to fill his lungs with air in the middle of an asthma attack. I shined the light across the floor and first saw his large blue feet; his extremities were very cyanosed, indicating a deficiency of oxygen in the blood. I played the light up his legs to his torso and then realized the rest of his body was sliding off the seat to the floor. He had been sitting upright in a chair trying to breathe and had either fallen asleep or gone unconscious.

"Sir? Can you try to slow your breathing down?" I felt his pulse and realized how weak it was and that help was needed beyond what I could do. "I'm going to start some oxygen with a mask and then get the doctor for you." I set the mask on his face and dashed out of the room to the nursing station to dial for an intern. That demonstrated a very good reason for those hourly checkups!

On a medical-surgical floor, most of the deaths took place in the middle of the night, with the darkness of the outside creating a fearsome atmosphere on the inside. Sunrise would still be a few hours away, and I had seen my share of horror movies. I was scared.

"Who wants to come with me? Come on, anyone, please. I hate the dark."

Often my classmates felt the same way, so we made the rounds together when possible. I didn't want to be alone, as I feared that I would find someone who had died.

Some patients became favourites, based on their personalities, friendliness, or lack of demands. I was often assigned to a four-bed ward to look after a young woman terminally ill with cancer. She was a few years older than me, and I could not imagine how it must have felt to be in her place as she suffered. I could not chat about my dates and other life experiences, as they were so terribly opposite of what her life had become. I would try to be upbeat and talk about easy subjects—the weather, the menu for the day—aimless words to fill in the silence as I did her personal care. I could tell by her pallor that she was in a fragile state, and as mealtime rolled around, I prepared to help her.

We started on the soup, and in the middle of a mouthful, her eyes flew open in a surprised look. I thought the liquid had gone down the wrong way. But there was no choking. Then I thought, *My gosh, she fainted!* I called her by name and gave her shoulder a gentle touch. No response. I grabbed the bedside buzzer, pressed it hard, ran out of the room to yell for help, and ran back in. In those few short moments, she had truly, soundlessly died. I stood by her bed, holding her hand tight in a state of complete shock, with tears rolling down my cheeks. One minute she was alive, the next minute she was not. A sensation of pins and needles descended over me as the room darkened in my sight. *Oh my God, what's happening to me? Am I dying too?* Overwhelmed and in shock, I felt my legs weaken. I grabbed the bedsheet as I started to slide down to the floor. By now other nurses had responded to my call for help. They pulled the bedside screens around her. The shared room was completely silent. The head nurse took one look at me and ordered me to go back to residence for one hour and said that senior staff would deal with this.

Competent and professional, she took charge, and I did what I was told. I left by the back stairs, not wanting to be seen in such a state. I went outside, crossed the courtyard, climbed the stairs to my room, and lay on my bed crying. I tried to gather my nerves so I could return to the ward and pretend all was well. I would never forget this sudden death, and I felt the emotional shock for a very long time. However, I was determined to stay with nursing, to get through the experience, and to not give up.

Death could and often did enter quietly, taking a life away without any fanfare or fuss after a long illness. I had been taught mortuary care, believe it or not. Discovering a dead patient meant noting the exact time of the event and ascertaining they truly were dead—no pulse felt, no heartbeat in the chest, no breathing attempts, no recordable blood pressure—and then a call to the intern or doctor to come and do the same check and confirm findings.

Rigor mortis would set in as the body temperature cooled. Students shared this care, as none of us wanted to be alone, closed in with a corpse, surrounded by curtains. There was nothing to relieve the tension of these moments, and no light chatter could ease the pressure. Here we were, kids really, carrying out these actions as if it were the most normal thing in the world. It was not. During a scene like this, my coping skills descended into the basement as a sense of dread and horror went through my mind.

What am I doing here? Is this what nursing is?
I'm out of here. I can't do this.

But I stayed.

Even so, self-doubt filled me. Sometimes I would imagine the person took a breath. "Is he coming alive again? Did you see that? His chest moved!" The other student would look wide-eyed at me, and then we would settle down to the task at hand, trying not to scare each other out of our wits. My imagination would race, my pulse would soar, my hands would shake. We could not leave the eyes open, or any limb bent, because it would be difficult later to straighten the body out for the coffin. So, we straightened limbs, closed eyelids, replaced sets of teeth, and then gave the body its final bath. Dressings, bandages, and all tubes had to be removed and disposed of.

I tried to distract myself by thinking about ancient Egyptian embalming. It's hard to imagine mortuary care being performed by a teenager, but that is what I had to do. Families had to be notified and given the opportunity to come into the hospital and say their goodbyes before the body was taken to the morgue. More reason for the final cleanup, the last hospital viewing. Then the paperwork and official forms were filled out by the attending doctor. If there was no last visit, we carefully shrouded the body, moved it to a mortuary trolley, and prepared to go to the morgue.

I closed all the ward doors, hoping no patient would see us rolling a shrouded body, and we took the stretcher down the hallway. An orderly accompanied us on this last journey. The morgue was not a place where we had very much experience, thankfully, and it was hidden away from public view, in the basement. It contained refrigerated, stainless-steel pull-out trolleys behind a refrigerator door. We tagged the body, transferred it into the unit, and tagged the door with the identification of the person. We didn't want a mix-up! If an autopsy were necessary, the body would remain in the morgue. Otherwise, the funeral home would be called, and morticians would arrive with their long black transport hearse. The exterior door was unmarked, but they all knew where to find it. Another transfer from the refrigerator to the vehicle.

I recall the challenge of finding a dead patient who had likely died before the previous round of checking. His son had been in for a quick visit, too quick for anything meaningful to take place, but no one really knows ahead of time that they are about to lose a parent. The elderly man had been in for surgery on a hernia, a simple procedure, but nothing can be taken for granted as to its outcome.

Had I missed seeing that he wasn't alive? Rigor mortis had commenced, and he was in a semi-seated position in bed. Rolling the bed flat did nothing to flatten his body; it wanted to stay bent in a sitting position. It took us several attempts to smooth him out, so to speak, placing heavy pressure on cold limbs at one end and cold shoulders at the other. It was a macabre moment, leading me to giggle inappropriately. Hysteria perhaps? A bad movie in which I played a role?

"Oh my God! Push harder." We pushed. "Yikes. This isn't going to be good when the day staff hear about it. Hold the feet and I'll push the shoulders."

I wondered if I should warm up a sheet and place it across his chest. Would that soften him up? I feared being taken to task if the head nurse found out that I had done rounds too late to discover he had died. A cause for being expelled? I discovered there was no way to warm up a cold body after death.

One could try to find something humorous in the image, but in truth there was nothing even remotely funny with the situation we found ourselves in that day, and many others. A bent corpse does not fit on a trolley or in a refrigerated unit, let alone a casket!

The hours flew by at night, and though the demands were different from the daytime, I was busy making rounds and answering the patients' buzzers for bedpans, urine testing, and pain relief. In between, as always, I had to check that all records were noted properly and that the cardex was up to date.

In comparison to today's age of rapid communication, computers, emails, cellphones, tweets, and voice mail, the system for patient information sharing in the 1960s was very basic. At the main desk of the nursing station, the wall featured numbered slots corresponding to each room on the floor. The chart held a complete collection of information about each person, an intern's history, a sheet of prescribed drug therapy data, vital stats on blood pressure, temp, and pulse, liquid intake and output if required, fresh sheets of paper for the doctors' notes at each visit, and his or her orders.

The front desk on the evening and night shifts was lit with lamps, not bright overhead lighting. One stepped off the elevator and saw a calm, quiet area, wherein order was the rule. The only well-lit space was the drug room, for obvious reasons. The subdued lighting gave a somewhat homey atmosphere of control and authority, with an "All is well" message, even when it was not.

One of our night-shift duties was the preparation of the blood testing tray for the morning lab technician. Students worked together, going through every patient chart, double-checking the doctors' orders for blood work, and then writing the requisition. On a large metal tray, we laid out the correct glass tube and syringe with its steel plunger and needle to draw the blood. The large bin, filled with a selection of syringes, was confusing. Each type had to correspond with the amount of blood for the test. Therefore, we had to know which one to choose or risk making a mistake. Some tubes were empty, others had an anticoagulant that would keep the blood from congealing.

Heaven help us if we made the wrong choice. When the lab technician arrived on the floor, she wanted to go from patient to patient in an efficient manner. We had labelled each tube in the early morning hours, and if something wasn't right, you were sent rushing to the desk to retrieve another tube or syringe. A "calling down" by the nurse in charge followed, and the next time the student did the blood tray in the middle of the night, it would be done to perfection—another learning-on-the-job moment. It would be many years into the future before this task was shifted to a central location where lab techs prepared their own tray.

After the lab technicians finished their work, we took the back copy of the requisition to the nursing station and filed each one with the chart, to be removed when the lab report came back.

Hospital patients fell into several categories. Those with no ability to pay shared a public ward with four to seven beds. There were semi-private rooms with two patients each, and a few private rooms available for those who had the money to pay the extra amount, wanting privacy and to be alone in their misery. Single rooms were also assigned to the very ill or those close to dying who needed intense attention from the nursing staff. There were no specialized intensive care units at the time, so a patient's condition, if it was progressively worsening, dictated a private space whenever possible. Visiting hours could be relaxed for the families of patients who were alone in a room, but long hours enclosed in a space looking at four walls was not an optimal experience for the human spirit.

I remember taking the time to visit an elderly lady in a solo room. She had no visitors and was always alone. She was waiting for a long-term nursing home bed, and none of her family visited or were able to take her home. I read the newspaper to her, and in that manner I kept up on current events. She was too ill to read a book. Waiting for God or a nursing home bed without any distraction would not be my first choice. I understood that families were well-intentioned when they paid for privacy, but the loneliness was unpleasant.

This patient's needs were very few. She was obviously wealthy because she wore beautiful sapphire and diamond rings on her thin fingers. Her jewellery was so loose, it could slip off and get lost in the bedding.

"Could I place a thin piece of tape in front of your rings? I'd hate to see them fall off and be lost." I mentioned my concern to the head nurse and suggested she have a conversation with my patient about having the family take responsibility for her jewels and sign them out of the hospital. I spent time with her over the next few days, as she was assigned to my care. At some point the family came in and removed her rings, but my patient still wanted to wear jewellery, albeit not five-carat stones. She settled on a small diamond ring and a solitaire green olivine ring in a Tiffany setting.

Finally, arrangements were made for her transfer to a nursing home, and she asked that "Miss McCarthy" visit her. The head nurse accompanied me to the bedside, curious as to why. The patient was sitting up in bed with a pretty pink bed jacket on. Her thin hair had been combed, and she looked at me with a smile.

"I want you to have my olivine ring, my dear, because you were right to tape my diamonds on my fingers and you cared about me."

With the head nurse present, I asked, "Is it okay to accept such a gift?" Given the sincere desire of the patient, I was allowed keep it. I would treasure it always.

Chapter 7

In JULY OF 1960, MY SISTER, SHIRLEY, GAVE BIRTH to her second daughter, Pamela. I was called to the case room (the obstetrical delivery room) and advised that my sister wanted me there, as Pamela had just been delivered. Sis had received a nitrous oxide mask to relieve her pain, and she seemed quite out of it, barely conscious. Her labour had been difficult, and she looked very pale and exhausted. This was the first time I entered the environs of the delivery room. What an impression it made on me. I had just missed the birth by a few minutes, but baby Pam was swaddled in warm blankets in an incubator, awaiting transfer to the nursery. I looked at her in amazement.

"Hi, sweet little girl, welcome to the world. I'm your auntie."

I took a quick glance around the delivery room and the equipment. Something spoke inside my heart, filled with feelings of joy and excitement for them both. At that very moment I knew case room nursing would be my special interest.

This is it! This is what I want to do when I graduate. I want to work here in obstetrics, and finally I know a good reason for staying in nursing.

I had to go on duty elsewhere but later walked over to the maternity floor. I entered what I thought was my sister's room to see the obstetrician and the resident frantically working on the patient to save her life. I thought I had entered the wrong room.

I didn't recognize my own sister. She had suffered a massive hemorrhage, with blood leaving her body faster than the two doctors were able to pump a transfusion into her. She was unresponsive, and all colour had drained from her face, leaving her lips blue. They didn't know it was my sis and yelled at me.

"We're going to lose her! Get in here, take over the resident's position. Pump the blood."

I took over pumping for the resident, squeezing the bag of blood by hand to force it to enter her vein faster than the intravenous could drip it. The resident tried to find another vein to start a third infusion.

Oh my God, don't die. You can't die. Don't . . .

It seemed to take forever before she rallied from their efforts, and I stood, shaking, by her bedside when the worst of the emergency was over.

"Sis? It's me. You're going to make it. Look at me, breathe deeply, hold my hand." It was all a jumble of thoughts as I tried to understand what I was seeing. There is a thin line between life and death, and my sister had stood at its edge. As she stabilized, the operating room was being prepared for her return for emergency surgery. This brief and near-tragic experience once more cemented in my mind that I wanted to study obstetrical nursing and specialize in it.

Before my first year finished, I moved from the fourth floor to make space for new students. I was assigned a room with its own sink in the more modern part of the residence. This was a huge improvement over the shared communal washroom. Where did those first twelve months go? Watching the new students arrive, it came as a shock that the probies weren't us! I was now an intermediate student. I had done an incredible amount of book work and gained invaluable practical experience. The steep learning curve of the first year was over. The mountain was ahead.

I chose a double room, and this meant having a roommate. Ann Louise Lewell and I lived side by side for a while. Sharing a room gave us a space twice the size of the old, and instead of metal bed frames, the furniture was made of red maple. Ann and I were friends, and we shared and whispered our private thoughts in the dark of the night after lights out. This arrangement lasted almost one year until my inability to sleep soundly put an end to it. I would come off night duty and go to bed wide awake, tossing and turning until mid-morning. If Ann came in at lunchtime I would wake up and be challenged to return to sleep. When her day shift ended, the door would quietly open, and I would be disturbed again. I couldn't in fairness expect her to live like a mole because of my problem. I worked a lot of night shifts, and every footstep in the hall outside my bedroom became a reason to toss and turn.

I moved into a single room again to save my sanity and to rest undisturbed with earplugs and eyeshades, along with recorded white noise. My biorhythms were definitely out of sync.

What kept me going in residence was my stack record player, my cribbage board, my books and magazines piled in the corners, my ability to whistle my way through most challenges, and my off-the-wall humour that helped me laugh at myself while others joined in. My repertoire of jokes expanded with each shift.

I tried to swim often at the local Y, even though the old gang of swim buddies and lifeguards had either moved on or away. According to my mom, I swam before I could even walk, no doubt due to the fact that I was ten pounds at birth and grew to be a bit of a beluga before I could stand up and walk around. Fat floats, and I was in the water very early!

In high school I had spent several hours a week learning to lifeguard, a feat that would come in handy at times when swimming in the Kennebecasis River and sailing from the Renforth dock. I was surprised in my second year of nursing to receive an invitation to coach a group of swimmers preparing for competition, and I jumped at the chance. It was necessary that I clear a schedule with my nursing superiors. To coach systematically and regularly before a competition meant I had to be able to commit to being there. My plan was to push the girls' team as hard as I could and to train them for endurance and speed.

They had to swim eighty-eight laps of the pool, working on the front crawl, the backstroke, and the breaststroke. I made them do deep breathing exercises, expanding their lungs so they could hold more air—the idea being more air in, the longer they could swim without needing to take a breath. Bilateral breathing was in the future, and I had never heard about it. Each time they practiced, I saw their emerging strength and I began to hope that, just maybe, they had a chance at winning. I fuelled them with sliced oranges soaked in honey, and it seemed to work, a supercharge of sugar energy to provide power for the event. We were to race at the same pool I had trained in, full of chlorine odours and happy memories.

From my diary, October 1, 1960

My girls won! by thirty-nine points and broke two speed records. St. Vincent's scored fifteen points, and Saint John High and Vocational tied with fourteen points. We took diving too.

Simple words that hide the fact that they had worked tremendously hard, and so had I, managing to swim and work and study. The newspaper published a picture of us all in the water holding the trophy. In the noise of the pool surroundings, the reporter misheard my name, so I was in the paper as Coach Nancy.

My efforts at exercise were defeated by my new-found fudge-making skills in the residence kitchen. I made pot after pot of brown sugar and peanut butter fudge.

Walking back to my room, satiated by four fat chunks of the sweet treat, I would announce in the hallway, "Fudge is in the kitchen, help yourself!" I don't know if I was being generous or just didn't want the fat on my hips.

The fudge went fast and then I would go down to the residence gym to shoot basketballs with a rather deflated ball, memories of my high school prowess fading fast with my solo hoop shots bouncing off the rim.

Organized exercise wasn't a top priority for the hospital despite it being a health-based organization, yet there was a recreation club in place to encourage badminton, ping-pong, volleyball, and basketball. Getting the right number of players together and meshing schedules was a challenge, and my shift work interfered constantly with my hopes for sport. Dashing around the wards, up and down the stairs, through the tunnel to the hospital, and back and forth to class was my workout.

I liked to whistle, and the habit got noticed. There was a superstition about whistling inside the hallowed walls of a hospital, which came to my attention when the head nurse took me aside and in no uncertain terms told me, "The whistling has to stop!"

And the reason is?

Had she looked into my eyes, she would have known exactly what I thought of her order. I couldn't answer, and I didn't know if I could obey.

My habit was about to be shut down, and my

subconscious struggled to get this across to my conscious brain. My puckered lips would just pop a tune out of my mouth, and I would be a few bars in before I would remember to shut up with a forced stop. I no longer sharpened my whistling ability on a popular tune, and for a while I moved my pursed lips in a silenced pucker.

Ultimately this too stopped, but to this day I still enjoy it, letting my whistle blast forth, with no adverse effects. Several of my classmates would later sign my yearbook pages with "I will miss your whistle!"

At the beginning of my second year, the uniform I wore with pride had a new attachment. A small bar pin, the red metal insignia of an intermediate student, was attached to my collar to mark the transition from first to second-year status. I had now passed one-third of the way through nursing, and where had the time gone? There was no great celebration for this moment. I simply walked down to the nursing office, picked up the pin, and attached it to my collar. I still wore black shoes and stockings, looking forward to the day when I would be rid of them permanently.

Out in the real world, away from the nurse's

uniform, a fashion change was rapidly taking place. Capri pants, shift dresses, pillbox hats, and the trending higher hemlines were accompanied by a general softening of the fashion rules of the former decade. Comfort was in, and men's styles also loosened up. The fellows began to sport longer hair and sideburns, wider ties, and a more relaxed style of clothing. Those of us who could afford new fashions bought them, even without the frequent opportunities to wear "outside" clothes. Remember the letter from Miss Stephenson? "You will not need as many clothes as you have previously."

While the fashion world was changing, the music world was exploding! Rock and roll, the staple of high school dances in the late fifties, was now taken over by pop singers, whose lyrics were aimed at the teenaged market of lovesick girls and young men dreaming of conquest. "I'm a Man," "Save the Last Dance for Me," "A Teenager in Love," "Will You Love Me Tomorrow," "Take Good Care of My Baby," "Stand By Me," and Roy Orbison's trio of spectacular hits—"Only The Lonely," "Crying," and "Oh, Pretty Woman"—played on radios and stack record players.

The big dance craze was the twist. Some of us judged this as too provocative and sexy, until the dance floor erupted in movement, then who could resist? Our uniforms did not keep pace with the fashion world, of course, and we continued along in aprons, with dresses thirteen inches from the floor.

I was about to take a two-week vacation but agreed to be part of an orientation and welcome night for the new students. Our class had to provide the skits and contribute to an evening of laughter for the newbies. I decided to take an old apron and paint it, borrowing it from another student, Ann Barbary, as mine were all in the laundry. I wrote large, fat letters, easily read from the audience, with an indelible ink pen. I chose the acronym SHITT. In small print underneath, I explained that SHITT stood for "Student Hopefuls in Training Tonight." I performed the skit with bedpans, wearing the decorated apron with its emblazoned SHITT in clear view. The apron was to retire to the garbage immediately after, but does anything ever go as planned? My first act was a roaring success as I walked around with a bedpan full of chocolate milk and marshmallows, pointing to the shocking word.

Wow! I really chose the right act to do!

I followed up with a lip-synched song and dance of Peggy Lee's famous hit, "Fever." The tune and lyrics were at the top of the charts. I lip-synched to the soundtrack and stood in front of the group, dancing and wiggling around. I wore a great curly white wig and a tight dress along with high heels. I had painted my lips red in an exaggerated bow, and my lids with blue eyeshadow.

I think you do this pretty good; you missed your calling. Smug little nursy, starting a new career for one night.

The new students and the old gave me uproarious applause and demanded an encore for which I was not prepared but muddled through.

Afterward, I had to visit a new student, Minte Chase, a best friend from high school. I explained I was heading out for two weeks, and I happily and ignorantly took off for vacation.

I promptly forgot about the apron. *Mea culpa.* Never assume that someone else will look after things, and sure enough, the owner of the desecrated apron did not pick it up. I have no idea who did the final cleaning of the auditorium that evening, but seeing an apron on the floor, it was bagged and sent to the laundry. All hell broke loose! The ink acronym did not wash out, and SHITT made its way to the administration office, and thence to the director. All our clothing had personal name tags, and Ann Barbery was the owner of the apron, despite not being the one who had done the deed. Staff in the laundry felt obligated to report the foul message on the apron. How easy it was to assume that Ann was guilty.

She was called in for questioning and told the director that she was not the guilty one. She was threatened with expulsion if she didn't own up to who had written the word on the sacred cloth. Ann, bless her, held fast and wouldn't admit that it was Francene McCarthy who wrote the offending word on the apron.

Ann phoned me at my home in Renforth, explaining the situation that was taking place in the administration office.

"Hi, Francene, we have a situation on our hands." She gave me the full description. "The apron went to the laundry by mistake."

"Whose mistake?" I asked.

"Well, I don't know, but Stephenson is going to expel me if you don't own up."

With those words my heart sank. I had visions of personal failure, expulsion, going to work in a restaurant, living at home forever. All flashed through my mind. I needed no convincing that the only correct action I could take was to call the director's office, book an appointment, and go in with my confession. I fully expected to be tossed out of the school of nursing. I dressed professionally in my student uniform and tried to look as remorseful as I felt.

Miss Stephenson was very grave. She sat rigidly upright, her bony hands folded in a tent-like position, forming a wall between us. She had the power, and I was a sweating mouse about to lose its head. I remember her words. "Miss McCarthy, I cannot believe it was you who did this. Your name never entered my mind."

I had the thought, *Who had she deemed could do this?*

I apologized for my actions, tried to explain about the acronym, which I could now see was so damn childish as to be pathetic. She let me go with just a warning, and I never again defaced a uniform.

The grapevine moves fast in a nursing school, and thus my classmates learned at once what the outcome was after I called Ann. She was relieved to hear from me.

"It's over, Ann. I saw the director and told the truth," I told her. "I guess honesty really is the best policy."

—∿—

My two-week vacation flew by and then it was back to training. I looked forward to community-based nursing with the Victorian Order of Nurses, the VON. As its name implied, it had begun in the reign of Queen Victoria who established it in Great Britain. I was ready to be out of the hospital environment after the SHITT incident.

It would be a brief respite from the hospital. This was a fun escape from the routine, and I wore a cute navy-blue uniform with a tight belt. The week's program included a day with Family Welfare and

Children's Aid, attendance at a tuberculosis clinic, and public health services.

The registered nurses who made up the VON made their daily rounds in all types of weather and circumstances, being the eyes of the hospital and the doctors. They were a dedicated, professional group of women who loved what they did and were loved in return. The work was challenging, dealing in the home with the chronically ill, post-surgery clients, people with diabetes, hypertension, asthma, and some just needing a bed bath from a nurse if families couldn't manage to do it. I recall going to the apartment of an elderly lady, and according to the records, she needed a weekly bath. I knocked at her door and there was no answer. I knocked again, same thing. Finally, I went to the next apartment and asked the resident if she knew the whereabouts of the old lady. She told me that my patient had left a few minutes before my scheduled visit. I walked down the stairs to the sidewalk and saw an elderly woman in a housecoat and I yelled her name. She took off at a good clip and I went after her. How could she move so fast? The street had side alleys running from it, and she knew the way better than I. I could not catch her in the end, and I had to report that I had not succeeded in locating her. Thus, she was bathless for another week.

Rain or shine, mostly on foot, we visited the

overcrowded slums of a section of Saint John. I became aware of the extent of the slums and grinding poverty.

Every apartment was owned by an absentee landlord who charged exorbitant rents while letting the buildings fall into disrepair. Built decades before, what formerly had been private three-storey homes were now divided up into tiny spaces and rooms. Inside the hallways there was an odour of urine, the smell of fried cooking, and garbage piled in the corners. Graffiti marked the walls, and lights were either burned out or dangled from cords. Every voice could be heard, and there was no privacy through the uninsulated rooms. The walls and corridors had not seen soap and water in a very long time.

What a stench! I'm going to stink when I get back to the residence.

I felt nervous while making the rounds with the nurse in charge. I had spent a year of my preteen life living in a slum, and I knew just how bad things could be in certain neighbourhoods.

I soon felt a different emotion. I was amazed that we were treated with absolute respect. We had nothing to fear, even in the most decrepit and filthy slums, and we were never subjected to foul language. Our nurse's uniform was our protective badge of honour, and in the lives of solitary and lonely people, we were the bright light in their day.

I have a vivid memory of a poignant case where we drove out toward the airport and turned off onto a dusty, unpaved road. A few desolate miles in, we came across what appeared to be an abandoned and boarded-up school bus. However, it was not. Inside, a mother took care of ten children, all different ages. None of them looked alike, due to different paternity.

The portable gas camp stove held one large pot of boiling potatoes and onions. This was to be shared by all of them together, after it cooled. It was eaten without spoons; they dug into the mash with their fingers.

This can't be real!

I was shocked by the squalor and filth of the children. Our visit was to determine if the impetigo on their faces was responding to treatment provided, and that as far as neglect went, they were not being starved or assaulted. Apart from the drying crusts of scabs around their mouths, they seemed in reasonable health, happy with their solo parent and the simplicity of the surroundings of the woods and nearby stream. They knew nothing else. I was literally speechless. The kids peered at me, and I peered at them.

Inside I was thinking, *Oh my God! Why is this allowed? She's out here with all these kids, no phone, no nothing.* I imagined the worst. It reminded me of the descriptions from a Charles Dickens novel. The mother appeared to be mentally challenged and had been servicing various men who found their way on the back road to the bus, thus the children resembled the mother in some way but were born to different fathers. This arrangement couldn't continue into the winter, and I knew, as did the VON, that an intervention would be done that would send the children in different directions to foster care.

When I finished my district nursing experience, I had no further follow-up with the people I met. In later years of my nursing career, I would see other examples of neglect and lack of a social response to the horrific conditions of families.

The short time spent away from the hospital was over too quickly, but it was a welcome change from the discipline and grind of training. All too soon it was back to the wards, but the memory of public nursing lasted a long time. I knew that the compassionate nurse who supervised me would continue to do what she could for the family in the bus.

I moved on to obstetrics, in particular the case room, where a significant part of our training took place during the second year. Pregnant mothers came to us in labour and were first admitted to the preparation room. The most essential action was to listen to the fetal heart, then take a brief history. To lower the risk of infection in the case of a surgical incision of the perineum, we had to shave the patients' perineal hair and the pubic area, preparing for a surgical episiotomy that was thought to be a better alternative than an accidental tear during delivery.

It was tough on the patient to be shaved, especially when in active labour with contractions coming every few minutes. This was followed by a soap suds enema, so the bowel would not empty during delivery. I was never sure if this was to help the mother or the delivery doctor. It had to be a wretched feeling, adding the cramps of an enema to labour pains, but cleanliness dictated the practice.

No one wanted this procedure, and often I would hear, "No! You don't really need to do this, do you?" It was stop-start action, as a contraction came, their faces screwed up in pain, and there was no holding still.

The delivery room had green tiled walls lined with equipment: an anaesthetic machine with its nitrous oxide and oxygen, cans of ether and masks; packages of forceps, only used during a difficult birth to apply traction on the baby's head to turn the fetus or to extract it from the birth canal; and stainless-steel tables covered in beige linens and sterile strings for tying off the umbilical cord. There were no plastic cord clips at that time. The delivery tray held scissors for cutting the cord, additional forceps to clip any bleeders (blood vessels that would not stop bleeding on their own), large basins for sterile water, and a suction cup and catheter for cleaning out the mucous from the newborn's airway. Syringes with their long needles were used to freeze the perineum if an episiotomy was needed. There was a large stainless-steel bowl used to hold the placenta after it was delivered.

I was taught to perform a rectal exam, learning to distinguish the feel of the cervix as it opened with the contractions and to note just how far it was dilating. This established the progress of labour and that those contractions were doing their job. I learned how to palpate the mother's belly and note how far down the fetal head had moved and whether the fetus was lying across the uterus in the transverse position. Sometimes the head did not move down because the baby was upside down, presenting in the bum-first position, known as a breech delivery.

Labour was hard work and contractions could be so painful that a patient would cry out and ask to be heavily sedated. The drug that relieved pain in the mother was rapidly transmitted into the baby's own blood supply. The relief was minimal.

I learned how to surgically scrub my hands and arms, preparing to assist in the case room. I loved the feeling of urgency and expectation, standing at the big scrub sink and lathering up along with the doctors. I gowned and gloved, then assisted the doctor to do the same.

Maternity care was hands-on in the 1960s. There was no digital or machine monitoring. Nurses sat with their patients during active labour, instructing them how to breathe deeply as the contraction reached its peak and how to relax between the pains and let go of tensed muscles.

"Breathe, breathe deeply, fill your belly, that's it, the contraction is at its peak, come on, breathe, and relax now as it wears off."

I used words of encouragement to talk to the mother and distract her through the pain. I held my hand on her belly, watching it tighten as the uterine muscle worked hard to push the baby down and out.

I monitored the fetal heart rate frequently, and if the amniotic sac of fluid surrounding the baby spontaneously ruptured, I observed its colour. If it changed from clear to greenish, it indicated a fetus was in distress, as the tinge came from meconium, baby poop, inside the uterus.

Compression on the umbilical cord caused distress by it either being twisted below the body, creating pressure and reduced oxygen flow, or looped around the baby's neck or against its chest.

The presence of bright red blood indicated that the afterbirth, or placenta, was separating prematurely from the wall of the uterus; complete separation would cause immediate death for the fetus and a high risk of death for the mother from blood loss. The incidence was rare. It needed a very rapid surgical response if there was to be any hope for the survival of the baby. The operating theatre had to be ready for a Caesarean section.

Without warning, an emergency could take place. A fetal heart could speed up too high or drop too low, out of the range of normal, and we shifted our routine speedily to intervention.

I recall my first time with such an event. Another student and I dashed down the corridor with the groaning patient on a stretcher, two students in a race against time.

"McCarthy, you scrub."

I did so alongside the surgeon. The circulating nurse had already removed the draperies on the tables, and I did the strategic things I had been taught to do. We began to quickly count all the sponges and instruments to be used in the operation. I tried not to look flustered, to appear competent. I prepared the suture materials, but I felt insecure. I feared making a mistake. Would I thread the wrong suture to the wrong needle? I never did screw up, but the possibility was on my mind.

Everyone will hear my pounding heart. I'm so excited! And scared!

Time counted, every second of it. The anaesthetist was present, managing the sedation at just the right moment of intervention so that the scalpel could begin its job in the hands of the obstetrician.

"Everybody ready?" he asked.

The surgeon made the first deep, rapid cut of the blade through the abdominal skin while the resident tied off bleeders and adjusted the retractors to provide a wider opening. He continued through the layers to the uterus. Emergency sections were messy, incising the tissues as fast as possible to extract the baby.

The fetus was still inside the protective sac of water, curled up and about to be delivered while the resident held the retractors on either side of the opening, pulling skin and muscle wider apart so the baby could emerge. It must have been a shock, one minute inside a warm, wet cocoon and the next, blinking in the glare of bright overhead lights.

What a sight! A live infant, screaming lustily, with a perfectly round head, as it had not been compressed in the trip down the birth canal.

Thank God. I likely should have been thinking, *Thank the doctors and the nurses*, whose timing worked together to get the infant out in a hurry.

The delivery room was a place of electric tension, as at any given moment something could change. My memories of the case room include the sense of mystery and urgency, the joys and the sorrows, the atmosphere, and the expectant fathers who paced in the waiting room and asked many questions. They were nervous as they listened to the strange sounds their wives made.

In that day, very few men wanted to be in the delivery room. However, the times were changing, and fathers began to accompany their wives to be present at the birth. While some were a great support, others passed out on the floor. Klunk! Another man bit the dust. They would come to, very embarrassed, and get on their feet again. That would mean looking after two patients, but the trend would continue to grow until it became the norm for fathers to be present in the delivery room.

It seems hard to believe now, but it was the students who were called upon to administer ether. If mid forceps had to be used, the patient had to be sedated enough not to react and risk a high tear inside the vagina.

I held the gauze mask in its wire frame above the patient's mouth and nose, and dribbled ether from a can.

"I'm going to hold a mask over your face, just above your mouth and nose," I would say. "I won't clamp it down, and the ether will stink. I want you to listen to me as I tell you to breathe deeply and slowly. You'll feel the room spinning, but it only takes a few breaths and you'll be asleep. Work with me, come on, you can do this."

The woman would start to lose consciousness, and it was at that point I clamped the mask down over her mouth and nose and administered more ether. I recall one doctor yelling at me to "Pour it on, girlie" as he struggled with the forceps. I didn't "pour it on"; I applied a small amount more, as in my opinion any more ether would have killed her. I covered this up by dripping the ice-cold ether over one side of my hand, holding the mask, fooling the doctor into thinking I was following his command. I reeked of fumes after the delivery. I truly hated the smell. It conjured memories of my childhood tonsillectomy, the mask being forced onto my young face, and the impending panic of smothering. That memory motivated me to be very calm and not clamp the mask on a patient too quickly.

The fetal pulse was affected by the trip down the birth canal. The labouring mother would scream out her last intense pains while I placed the stethoscope on her belly to listen to the heart rate. I had to strap the patients' hands down so they couldn't contaminate the sterile drapes; the moms would grip the delivery table handles, pulling against them for added pushing power.

"Push, push, push."

The gush of amniotic fluid and blood accompanied

the smells, the sounds, and the smooth emergence of the baby into the brightly lit world outside the uterus.

I always marvelled at the first lusty cries, the blinking eyes, and the wee face all trying to register its world. The newborn, coated in a cheesy film, bloodied from the birth, was the most beautiful sight. I unstrapped the mother's hands so she could touch her baby when I laid it across her chest.

I noted the exact time of birth and the newborn's weight and length, counted fingers and toes, observed the palate of the mouth to make sure it was intact, and then inspected the baby's back to determine whether there was any evidence of a malformation such as spina bifida. I examined the head and fontanelle (the soft spot at the top of the infant's head where the bones of the skull have not yet grown together), placed silver nitrate drops in the eyes, and swaddled the baby in warm blankets. The practice of using silver nitrate drops had been in use for decades. It was to prevent infection from a sexually transmitted disease and was a standard of the day. Decades later the silver nitrate drops were discontinued but were followed by the use of an antibiotic drop in their place.

There were buckets of plastic alphabet beads to be threaded onto a tiny identification bracelet. It contained pertinent information, pink beads for a girl and blue beads for a boy, with the mother's surname. All of us students crafted bracelets for ourselves or made bookmarks from them.

Attention shifted from the birth as we waited for the arrival of the placenta. The doctor would observe the dangling umbilical cord as it lengthened and the uterus contracted powerfully to expel the bulky, liver-like tissue. I injected a drug called ergotamine into the mother's vein to contract the uterus. The doctor examined the tissue to make sure that it was intact, as fragments left inside could lead to a life-threatening hemorrhage.

I placed the newborn in a warm incubator for transfer to the nursery. I cleaned the mother from the after-effects of the birth, combed her hair, transferred her to a trolley, reunited her with her husband, and took her to the maternity ward where her care was handed off to the floor nurses.

They would closely monitor her blood pressure, pulse rate, and the state of the contracted uterus to observe for pending bleeds.

We said our goodbyes, then it was back to the case room. We cleaned everything used, scrubbed the floor, removed all the instruments to the dirty utility room, washed them, and rinsed the bloodied linen squares under running water before sending them to the laundry room. A student's work was never really done. Jill of all trades!

Most of the time in the delivery room, it was a

joyous occasion. That was the norm, thank good-
ness, but the reality also included times of loss
and sorrow.

Occasionally a spontaneous abortion, better
known as a miscarriage, would take place early in a
pregnancy. With the mother admitted in labour, an
effort would be made to slow or stop the contractions. Nature would take its course, and the outcome
was never assured. Newborns with a birth weight of
two pounds or less stood little chance of survival.
Despite the tiny size, a two-pound fetus appeared
fully formed, just in miniature. There was no way to
know the fetal weight in advance, as the technology
of ultrasound was far in the future.

I recall the following event with acute clarity. A
young woman, thought to be three to four months
pregnant, came in with a spontaneous abortion
in progress. The stainless-steel bowl was ready to
receive the slippery mass as it came away from her
body. She delivered an early *conceptus* (a Latin word
for a fetus at the very early stage of pregnancy), and
it didn't look human at all. The doctor covered the
bowl with a green cloth and handed it to me. "Take it
to the utility room." He didn't want to show the contents to the mother, as it looked mostly like mucous.

I admit to being curious as I carried the draped
container out of the delivery room. So, I looked
inside, under the cover.

The conceptus was a translucent glob of cells, and to my shock and amazement, in its centre was a rapid, frantic heartbeat. The tiny mass was the very essence of life itself, heart fluttering wildly in its last effort to stay alive but slowly losing the battle. Tears stung my eyes as I watched, with thoughts racing through my head about birth, life, death, and emotional pain all jumbled together in my nineteen-year-old, immature self. I sat on a stool, awaiting the moment when the heartbeat would slow and stop. At the start of our case room training, students were told that in the event of a dire emergency with a newborn baby, we could baptize the infant with the permission of the mother. This would be an extremely rare occurrence, and if the attending nurse was not a Christian, it could not be performed by her.

The beating heart did not look like a newborn. I took no time away to seek the okay. I baptized it, although I couldn't say "the baby." With deep reverence and sorrow, I spoke the words, "I baptize you in the name of the Father, the Son, and the Holy Spirit." In a fraction of a second, a brief brush with the Eternal swept across my mind. I held the bowl in my hands, looking down at it, while my tears fell. An eternity passed in a few minutes.

The memory of that moment never left me.

Chapter 8

STUDENT NURSES KNEW THE RULES. WE HAD heard them often enough. We were not allowed to marry during training. If anyone became pregnant and it was found out, the student would be immediately expelled. No exceptions were made, but I recall one example of the sad circumstance of a senior student expelled two months before the conclusion of her three-year training program.

She had tried very hard to keep the pregnancy hidden, by wearing a tight girdle, and to keep her weight gain to a minimum. But sadly, the obvious became known to the administration and she was expelled immediately.

Word travelled throughout the student body like wildfire, and we were angry with the rules and the sad fact that an excellent nurse was being tossed overboard. There were many upset students, furious that a promising career was cut off, sad for the student, sad for the fetus girdled so tightly, but most of all fed up with an administration so rigidly stuck in the past.

One afternoon, a few weeks later, I went on duty to a strangely tense and subdued atmosphere. The glass panel of the delivery room door was covered over with a paper, a birth was in progress, and I was ordered not to enter the room.

What the hell?

Ultimately this too became a secret that couldn't be kept. A third-year student was in premature labour. Her early pregnancy had gone undetected, labour had started, and no fetal heart had been heard. A dead fetus was anticipated, and there was to be an attempt to keep this all a secret and her delivery not to be disclosed. How this could take place was yet to be worked out.

The birth occurred and a very tiny baby was born, with no movement or first breath. It was placed in a bowl and covered with a green drape. The medical staff attended to the placenta and the patient follow-up.

Suddenly a tiny mewling cry emerged from the draped basin, and all hell broke loose. I only know the details because I was allowed into the delivery room after the fact, after the first sounds of life were heard from a very determined preemie wanting to live. Attention shifted immediately to the baby, the suctioning, warm blankets, the baby's weight, the call for a pediatrician, and the arrival of a special incubator.

I attended to the care of the student as she lay silent, tears coming down her face. She watched the efforts of all the medical staff working to save her infant. The miracle of this rough beginning to life was the amazing resilience of one of the tiniest babies ever born to survive in the General Hospital, to thrive and ultimately go home with its mother. Goodbye to nursing studies, hello to motherhood.

This type of surprise did take place sometimes. Even though a fetal heartbeat could not be heard, a live baby would emerge. A tiny fetus could be tucked under its sibling and instead of one baby, two would be born! A woman could carry two small babies equal to the weight of one large one, and I recall the surprise of being the person to detect twins just at the point of delivery.

I listened to the heart, and I listened again and then held up my hand with two fingers waving as I continued with the stethoscope on the mother's abdomen. The doctor looked at me in disbelief. Sure enough, two distinct and different heartbeats.

"We have a surprise for you; you're having two babies," the doctor announced.

Often, a mother would arrive on the verge of delivery and no doctor would be present. I did the best I could on these occasions, but I wanted to know more in case I had to be the one doing the delivery. On a momentous day for me, this is exactly what happened. As I was about to deliver the fetus, without an intern or obstetrician, the doctor rushed, ungloved, through the door and I looked at him, expecting him to take over.

"No, you're doing a great job."

He's confident. I'm not!

I could see the crown of the head, ready to birth.

"Check for the cord around the baby's neck," the doctor reminded me.

I inserted my fingers gently inside to make sure there was no evidence of the umbilical cord.

"There's no cord, it's okay."

Then I supported the perineum so it would remain intact as the baby came out. I did as he instructed.

"Stop pushing now, just pant, I want the baby to come out slowly," I instructed the mother.

It seemed to take forever, but only a minute went by as the mother panted, her perineum stretched, and I managed to grab a sterile towel to wrap the baby's shoulders as it slid out. A baby girl, in my hands. I had no idea how slippery a newborn was in the first few seconds. God forbid that it should land on the floor.

I did it! I delivered her baby, and it feels so amazing to do this! I hope I get a chance again, it's glorious!

The doctor grinned at me. "See? You're a natural!"

The memory of my earlier desire to be a doctor flooded my brain, a moment of looking back, but now I was looking forward.

After delivery, all mothers were transferred to the postpartum unit where they received immediate close attention; their pulse and blood pressure were monitored every fifteen minutes, and the top part of the uterus, the fundus, was measured to make sure it was staying contracted and expelling any blood gathering inside. I would determine this by noting how many finger widths below the belly button it could be felt. The assessments continued every fifteen minutes for two hours until it was deemed all was stable, then less frequently after that. Women stayed in the hospital for five to seven days or longer if there were complications or if they had delivered by Caesarean. Those few days in hospital were sometimes the only break a busy mother ever got.

Each patient had perineal care given daily. The episiotomy and vaginal discharge were observed for signs of infection. If stitches were reddened, a heat lamp was placed in the bed to facilitate healing.

Believe it or not, the student's job included the care of the bathrooms. No cleaning staff ran around to pick up soiled pads. I had to make sure there were enough sanitary napkins and that the used and soiled ones were placed in the large, often overflowing paper bag in the bin. It was a job I hated, seeing a filled bin and all the rest of the bloodied pads thrown on the floor, waiting for me to pick them up and clean up the mess. *Do they think I'm their maid?* In a multi-bed ward, the sweetish stink of blood filled the air, the downside of obstetrical nursing. If the toilet seat or the floor got dripped on, and it often did, I cleaned it up.

I'm a nurse and a cleaning woman combined.
Stop the grumbling, brain, and just do it.

Mothers who breastfed were actively encouraged and supported by the staff. The obvious question was, "Why would you want to get out of bed in the middle of the night and warm up a bottle when all you have to do is place your nipple in the baby's mouth and let nature do its thing?" Not always a convincing point, however, and not all moms agreed. Non-breastfeeding women suffered through engorged and rock-hard mammary glands, swollen with unused milk coming in. They were given an injection to stop lactation, and their breasts were tightly banded with strips of linen wound around front and back, a girdle of sorts, snug enough to stop the flow of milk and worn like a high-placed corset.

Nature meant breastfeeding to be easy, but it was not always the case. The initial pre-milk, called colostrum, caused the babies to pucker up their lips at its taste and scowl their faces. Latching on to an abundantly producing nipple was no mean feat. I helped the mothers, asking them to brush their baby's cheek with their nipple, while pressing two fingers on either side to get it to protrude and making sure the infant's tongue was in the right position. A hungry baby can bobble its head around in a rooting search, trying its darndest to get latched on.

Successful feeding assured the newborn a supply of the mother's own antibodies, protection against infection. Rarely, an abscess would occur when the milk ducts were unable to completely empty, and painful swelling would result. Hot packs were applied, and the milk was pumped out. Infection was treated with antibiotics, and if pain relief was needed, medication was given in small amounts due to the fact that it passed through the milk and into the baby at feeding time.

Most mothers had great success and went home to feed their infants the natural way without the bother of preparing formula and sterilizing bottles, let alone the cost of store-bought formula.

My work on the postpartum floor was followed by working in the neonatal unit. Part of the training in obstetrics included a stint here, where the care of underweight, premature infants in incubators, with all the attendant care of oxygen and intravenous tubes hooked up to fluids, took place. Tiny preemies also received formula feeding in very small amounts, with this being done by reaching into the incubator and gently handling the baby.

In the newborn nursery, an endless round of bathing and diapering was the norm. On the night shift, babies were held back from their mothers for the 2:00 a.m. feeding, and our task seemed to never end. A room full of crying, hungry, red-faced babies was a sight to behold and a racket to hear. New moms had the middle of the night to themselves in an attempt to encourage their babies to sleep through, a vain expectation, for infants less than ten pounds in weight were not ready to miss a feeding. Like clockwork, the babies wailed every three to four hours, and the sound could out-decibel a siren. Often the nurseries were full, with too few nurses to do the job without rushing. If the case room wasn't busy, a call would go out for their students to help.

The first early morning feeding on the wards was done by the mothers. The infants were delivered in a batch process on a rolling cart filled with the sound of howling. They would all be awake and ready, a steady uproar coming from their tiny lungs, and the sound magnified off the metal walls of the elevator.

Whenever I worked the night shift, I had serious sleep disruption with repeated dreams of crying babies and poopy diapers. There were no disposable nappies, and each one, once removed, was given a quick rinse in cold water before being bagged and sent down the laundry chute. If the smelly whoosh of hot air coming back in my face from the chute was any indication, pity the staff at the other end!

Postpartum depression, a serious mental health issue, could be triggered by the birth. It was not readily recognized by doctors or the families of new mothers. Sometimes in the presence of sleep deprivation, frequent feedings, and fussy babies, new moms would become exhausted and depressed. While exhaustion was normal, it could progress to an abnormal state of weeping and anxiety. The upheaval of female hormones combined with a lack of sleep could go on for months after delivery. Good family support with the nighttime feeding would allow the mother to catch up on rest.

Single mothers with very little support systems had it the worst. Today much is known about post-partum blues, as it used to be called, and timely intervention is a must. Without it, the outcome could be tragic. I still remember the phone call from a friend's family, six weeks after the birth of her baby boy. She had been severely depressed and went untreated. She hanged herself in the basement. I reeled in shock and felt the heartbreak of her family as we talked. An unthinkable tragedy, leaving a beautiful son without his mother.

I didn't want to leave the obstetrical unit, but leave I did as my education progressed. I was assigned to pediatrics on the eighth floor of the hospital. The legend of a ghost named Mary intrigued me. While I never saw it, I sometimes had the shivers as a cold draft passed by without explanation. If there was a spirit around, this could be the place.

Peds was housed in the old 1930s section of the hospital, and the units were separated by glass-topped cubicles. Miss Stanley was the elderly head nurse. Tiny, feisty, knowledgeable, and about to make us into excellent caregivers, she ran a tight ship.

The unit had a peculiar smell, a mix of urine, poop, vomit, feedings, and a general odoriferous air from the children. The first impression, apart from the smells, was how scared the kids must have felt in the cribs and beds, away from their families, amongst strangers. Parents had no special visiting privileges here. We looked after the routine procedures after surgery for tonsillectomies, broken and cast bones, and other more challenging post-operative care, such as for a cleft palate.

The long-term care of children with neurological disorders was typically not part of a young student nurse's past experiences, so they had no idea what to expect. These were inoperable conditions in the 1960s, and babies were maintained in the unit until their death. Those born with spina bifida, in which the base of the spine protruded on the outside of the skin, and tiny-headed microcephalic infants, born with little brain material inside the skull, awaited their sad passing.

Most devastating to me were the babies with hydrocephalus. The abnormal circulation pattern of cerebral spinal fluid resulted in grossly enlarged heads that destroyed normal brain function. There was no surgical intervention and no ability to perform a shunt. These children didn't die quickly. Their heads grew to massive proportions and filled up the width of the crib so that the skin touched both sides of the rails.

Our duty was to clean, diaper, and bottle-feed them and to turn them from side to side every few hours so that the skin didn't break down. It took two students to lift and safely position the head, and the child's eyes would rapidly dart back and forth and roll up into the top of the lid, giving the impression of looking at us. I was told they had no brain function left after all the massive compression caused by the swelling, but who really knew? Were there other compensating senses?

I never saw parents visit these babies, and at the end of my shift I stayed to hold their hands and sing a few lullabies. I was profoundly sad to see them waiting for death, and perhaps singing to them was actually to comfort myself. It all felt so unreal, babies and toddlers who could not toddle and never would, waiting to die in a crib.

I often worked the night shift with one other student, and we struggled to meet the demands of the children who were restless and crying to go home, and we made sure we had everything correctly prepared for the morning nurses. The same demands as on other floors were here too—preparing blood trays for the lab, getting urine samples, administering pain medication—except it was all for little ones.

We grew tired in the night, and around five in the morning we played the radio at the nurses' station with the sound cranked up, trying to keep awake with the early morning talk show and music.

Eventually my time on pediatrics ended. I had suffered emotionally with this experience, and the reality was, nothing could prepare a young student for the devastation of a child's pain.

Students had the opportunity to join Nurses Christian Fellowship. They met once a week for sing-songs, Bible study, and discussion. Miss Lois Floyd, RN, was the leader and sponsor of this activity, and she was well respected. Sunday night vespers were a part of the fellowship and offered a quiet winding down of the day. The participating students had summer fun together along with outings and devotionals. Religion had been forced on me at an early age, and it was enough to keep me absent from the fellowship. Even though I saw there were benefits in belonging, I stayed away with stubborn resistance.

That said, I knew that the New Testament urges each of us to love one's neighbour. There are many ways to do so, and I approached several of my classmates to join me in supporting the adoption of a young Italian boy through Foster Parents Plan. Each month I collected one dollar each from twenty of us to support Constantinople Piras. This was more than the required fifteen dollars, so we were able to provide a few extra items for Constantinople. Our biggest gift to him was a leather soccer ball sent to him in Nardò, Italy.

The foster mothers who supported this endeavour were Marilyn Bates, Diane Bovaird, Peggy Blenkhorn, Minte Chase, Nancy Everett, Diane Geldart, Lois Herbert, Pat Jardine, Anne Lewell, Lois Lingley, Avis Macdonald, Carol Montgomery, Norma Munroe, Carolyn Neill, Margie Patterson, Pat Pettifer, Jane Ross, Carol Reid, Sue MacKay, and me. I wrote short letters to the boy, to keep in touch, but our fostering of him concluded when our student days ended.

I continued with my prayers and Bible reading on my own. I felt more spiritual without being a follower of a regular church routine, yet when I had rare Sundays off, I went home to Renforth and attended the tiny Anglican church. I know upon reflection that I missed out on times of inspiration and friendship with other students.

I've always believed in life after death, and thus it is that I share a diary entry with you that reinforced this belief.

From my diary, June 24, 1960

Tonight, I worked the evening shift. My patient was Miss Wayne. She is quite elderly and always happy and in a big-hearted mood. Her mind is sensible and not prone to roam at all. I was in to rub her back at 9:30, and she was, as usual, charming. She made fun of the fact that she was single and referred to the widowed patient across the hall who ties flies for fishing as his hobby. She joked she might chase him until she caught him by the fly. We exchanged a few more pleasant remarks, and I finished the care of her roommate and turned out the lights for nighttime. I had entered the next room when I became aware of the bell ringing in Miss Wayne's room. She had taken a bad turn and the other patient went up to the desk at the nurse's station for help. Miss Wayne didn't appear to be breathing. The interns were summoned and two responded, determining that she still had a heartbeat. They ordered oxygen by mask, and I held it over her face. She returned to consciousness and said, "It's so dark! It was so dark. And Mother is waiting, standing there in a dress. She visited me and said, 'I have waited so long for you.'"

I believe she experienced a moment of death. I believe her soul saw Heaven, for the split fraction of a second just out of reach of life and not in the void of death. She had a brief period away from us, an infinitesimal moment. This has happened in operating theatres, in hospital beds, in drowning cases.

The ambulance bay was off limits to students. With siren blaring, lights flashing, the two-man crew would leave in their shiny vehicle to help or retrieve someone from any number of accidents or life-threatening situations. The service was effective and would result in a flurry of preparation in emergency, awaiting their return with their human cargo. I wanted to explore the ambulance and hide in it. This inclination toward such reckless behaviour had persisted all through my growing up, a desire to push back boundaries to see what I could find, while at the same time flaunting authority in not too obvious a manner.

I'm not sure what it said about me, but I didn't respect limits. I wanted to experience the rush of the ambulance and the noise of the siren wailing through the streets. I convinced another student to get in on the stunt with me. Neither of us gave any thought to the consequences of being caught or how we would return to the hospital after we jumped out of the vehicle at its destination point. Just at the end of our shift, an opportunity presented itself for this adventure. The call came in for the crew to get to an emergency, and we sneaked into the back of the vehicle. We bumped along in the rear of the ambulance and finally came to a screeching halt.

We assumed the rear cargo door wouldn't be opened until the patient had been assessed, but we soon found out we were wrong. We hadn't noticed the attendant's bag in the back of the vehicle. We'd given no thought to anything like the door being opened on arrival to retrieve the medical kit. Our discovery was imminent. The two responders were there at the rear door, and the jig was up.

"What the hell! Get out, now! We'll put you to work!"

Our silly, joking manner was quickly replaced by the seriousness of the situation, and we rapidly followed the two men into the building and up a flight of stairs.

Saint John had entire areas of decaying wood tenement buildings, divided up into different spaces for people to rent. Most were considered fire traps. The exterior of the buildings was weathered, a dirty grey after years of neglect, with shingles and clapboards covered in peeling chunks of old paint. They slouched on stone foundations riddled with gaps where the city's rodent population came and went. Stray cats added to the bleak look, and decades of cooking without ventilation gave a permanent smell of cabbage and fried food that cloaked the air. The forlorn look of the dwelling as we entered mingled with the eye-watering odour of urine in the halls.

The apartment door was open, and we were greeted by an elderly lady, who was crying.

"He's inside, in the bathroom," she said and ushered us into the apartment.

Looking over her shoulder, we all saw the bathroom door was wedged open by a man lying on the floor. His thin, elderly, and very blue body was stretched out of the tub, while his legs extended over the rim.

I whispered to my friend, "Is he alive, do you think?"

Not much chance of it, given his colour. He was very dead. His poor wife got on the phone to call someone with her awful news, and we could hear her saying, "No, I'm not alone, there are two sweet nurses here to stay with me."

I had visions of hours ticking by with her and a dead man, and what started as a juvenile lark now had looming implications for my future. The more pressing reality was that someone lay dead on the bathroom floor at the end of what we thought would be a fun experience! We boiled water in the tiny kitchen and made a pot of tea, while the ambulance attendants did the paperwork. I was never certain why tea was a comfort, but when all else fails and small talk is not in order, tea is taken.

We sat with his wife, perched on the edge of our chairs, wanting to bolt. She was comforted by the distraction of us being there, and thus some small, good purpose was served. The attendants removed the man's body from its tight squeeze in the bathroom and laid it atop a shroud placed on the bed. They tagged his foot with his vital statistics and then wrapped him in the cloth. They lifted him onto the stretcher and manoeuvred it down the stairs to the waiting ambulance, surrounded by nosy, onlooking neighbours. We said our sober goodbyes to his wife in a more serious mood than when we arrived outside her building. Her husband was about to start on his final ride, first to the morgue for an autopsy, then to the funeral parlour. Since there was no need for the upfront emergency responder to ride in the back, my friend and I squeezed in with the wrapped body. By some luck of the draw, we were never reported for this stupid indiscretion, the staff no doubt believing we had learned a lesson. Trust me, our joyriding in the back of an ambulance never happened again.

The emergency service was located on the main floor

of the hospital, combined with the outpatient clinics and the ambulance bay at the far end. It served as all emergency departments do today, but without the benefit of a formal triage. A flow of accident victims, people with fractures, lacerations, bites, stinging insect allergic reactions, surgical emergencies, sick kids, high temperatures, heart attacks, and obstructions came through the door. If you could name it, it happened.

I didn't spend much time there, but some of my classmates loved the experience for the sheer never knowing what would happen. If the unit was reasonably quiet, the first thing a student did was go into each room and check the supplies, making sure all was ready. Dressing trays, gloves, and bandages, all the sundry equipment had to be in an excellent state of preparedness. The student assisted the nurse in charge with the initial assessment of the patient, and, without calling it triage, those who needed attention first were prioritized. The interns also assisted with procedures, and when they were new on the service, fresh from medical classes, we would give them a little test and ask them to go to the seventh floor to find Fallopian tubes. Sometimes they fell for it and took off, returning with a sheepish look.

Children who suffered awful bike accidents would be brought in by crying parents and hysterical siblings. On one shift, a young boy on his bike had been hit by a car, and on impact, the bike's handle-bars had connected with his abdomen. He lay white and unconscious with no obvious wound, no head injury, yet here he was with his life ebbing fast. We clustered at his side, monitoring his pulse and blood pressure as it skipped and weakened. It was obvious that nothing could be done to alter the outcome as we tried to stabilize him, and I, along with everyone at his side, felt helpless. His pallor worsened. There was a sudden rush of bright red blood, flooding through the bed linens, and a collective gasp came from us, knowing he was dying. Any sense of hope now disappeared. An artery had torn inside his gut, and he was gone a few tragic moments later. We all were in tears. The doctor, ashen-faced, had the horrible job of letting the parents know. They must have known when they saw his face, as their screams and sobs travelled back to us. These tragedies never leave one's memory, so great is the impact.

The outpatient clinics were conducted in the day-time, in one section of the emergency department. Women with cervical cancer were treated with the insertion of uranium seeds, and at no time did anyone address the risk to our young ovaries when we worked in the vicinity of the radiation being given.

The equipment was sorely outdated and sometimes inoperative. My friend Donna witnessed first-hand the failure of the electrocautery machine. The patient was sedated, with her legs up in stirrups, about to undergo cervical cautery. The doctor inserted the speculum and began to burn off the tiny diseased tissues. There was a spluttering sound and a little puff of smoke wafted from the vagina just as the wiring failed. Donna was not an electrician, but with a patient sedated and at the ready, the procedure had to be done.

"Fix it," the doctor barked. She innocently looked at him and wiggled a few wires, not expecting that her questionable electrician skills would work. By some miracle of wire jiggling, the cautery tip glowed red and the intervention succeeded. As the tissue was treated, smoke began to billow out and, at the head of the table, the anaesthetist began to hum. Thinking to amuse us all, he sang the words to the song "Smoke Gets in Your Eyes."

Was I confident in the emergency department? Yes, for routine things, but life-threatening moments unnerved me totally.

I want out of here as soon as I can do it, just let me not screw up. Why do I feel insecure? I'm afraid of making a mistake. No one promised anything would ever be easy. What had I expected?

What is it about a challenge that forces one to

master it despite the associated risk? I grew up wanting to prove myself. To take risks. The courage I had as a risk taker was the courage I needed to summon in nursing.

As a young girl, the huge pine trees in the vicinity of my home drew me like a magnet. I climbed branch by lateral branch to the highest and thinnest of the limbs that could hold me, until they started to creak a warning. Then and only then did my brain say stop. I would dangle upside down, high above the forest floor, until the rush of blood to my head blurred my eyes and I would position myself upright again for the climb back to earth.

Later in my teen years it was the challenge of scaling the Minister's Face on the Kennebecasis River, with two school chums, in the dead of winter. The massive escarpment was coated with a thick, glossy buildup of ice. We did it on a dare after skating across the river with others, and many hours later we were alive to tell the tale. The Minister's Face was a difficult winter climb for professionals with all their equipment, but I did it with the aid of my toe picks and the two friends struggling with me.

As I matured, I took fewer chances and restricted my toehold ascents to the gravel pit walls in the old quarry in Renforth and Torryburn. A hidden ravine was a routine challenge that took my breath away with each effort. I climbed here with my high school friend Jane.

It's no surprise that in nursing, opportunities to explore and climb didn't exist. But I still needed to take risks and demanded it of myself. I settled on a plan to climb up the inside of the hospital dome. It was the crowning cap of the building, an illuminated landmark with a warning light at its top for aircraft navigational purposes. Its height out-soared many a city church spire, and it was absolutely forbidden territory for anybody except those with a security badge.

I began my preliminary scouting after my evening shift ended. Large warning signs were posted inside the narrow entryway, and high-voltage wires were attached to the walls, cabled together and humming with all the power that ran the entire hospital. I had to find out if any of the maintenance staff were around and if there was any way I could get past the signs and explore the space. If I wore my regular clothes it would be obvious that I was up to something, so I made the early decision to be in uniform if the opportunity came. I prayed I wouldn't see a nursing supervisor making rounds.

I knew after a few weeks of surreptitious exploration that the likelihood of anyone being near the place was very slim. I mentally accepted that I would do this. Much like the ambulance adventure, I gave no thought to risk. I was driven. What would be up there? What might I find? This was to be a solo exploration, and there was an element of wanting to overcome my own personal fears about being alone, in the dark. Much of this stemmed from early childhood neglect in a dysfunctional family, and I had the desire to flout the authority vested in the sign. Not liking imposed rules and wanting to test limits, I had an impulsive streak and was determined to prove I could do it. It would probably take a psychologist to fully understand my motivation.

The dome was difficult to access, but after a few forays into its upper regions, I located a metal staircase and closed door. I opened this with caution. A steel ladder was positioned up the brick wall, and at its top, another small door. I nervously began the ascent, with the immediate realization that my long apron was a hindrance to safely positioning each foot, so I hitched it up into my waistband. My black service shoes stood me in good stead and rung by rung I made my way up.

Don't look down. Don't look left or right. Just face the wall and keep going. My hands are sweating.

At the very top of the ascent, in front of my face, was a narrow opening to another door. I freed one hand to unlatch it and, with one final effort, heaved myself over the top and through.

Oh my God! I did it. I'm an idiot, but so what.

Surrounded by cables, metal ducts, air vents, pipes, and a range of different sounds, my heart raced. In the dim light, I could see it all. The space was hot, intensifying my sweat from the effort of climbing, and I looked around once more. Having met my goal, I didn't plan on staying for any length of time. An anticlimax for sure after all the planning and expectation. But how often do expectations get met? The atmosphere hummed and throbbed as I got on my knees and positioned myself backwards for the return.

Holy crap. Now I've got to get back down.

My imagination went wild, and I pictured a hand reaching out to grab me. My nervous Nellie thoughts took over.

I knew I would have a heck of a challenge going down if I slipped and hurt an ankle. Through my brain flashed the not-so-funny picture of me dangling on the ladder, which gave me a jolt of anxiety.

I was more scared going down than up, my damp fingers clutching the ladder with the full knowledge that it would be a long time before I was found if I had an accident. I made my way down, perspiring buckets, black-shod feet finding each rung with great precision. I had seen the dome from the inside and would not share that adventure with anyone. I walked back to the residence in my soiled uniform, with a sense of pride that I had pulled this off, and prepared to go to bed with my secret. My mind nattered at me, not ready to let go of the memory of the evening and full of questions about the why of it all.

This really was stupid, Francene. What did you get out of this?

No answer, and at last, sleep overtook me.

Chapter 9

IN THE INTEREST OF HISTORY, I SHALL DIGRESS from nursing. Briefly. You will understand why as you read along.

Saint John had two large competing department stores, MRA's (Manchester, Robertson, and Allison's) and Calp's. The first store was the one my mother worked in, and I got to know it well. The second was the competitor and held an annual fashion show in the nurses' residence.

MRA's was the leading department store in the city, and within its walls and halls one could find hats, gloves, suits, skirts, sweaters, dresses, petticoats, coats and outerwear, shorts and blouses, shoes, swimwear, high-fashion labels, wedding dresses, formal wear, menswear, children's and infant wear, furniture, silver, bone china, crystal, and sports equipment. In my memory the store was the Selfridges of Saint John! As Great Britain emerged from Victorian times in the early twentieth century, a new model of clothing store took shape, one in which women could order clothes fully made up and purchased off the rack—much as we do today. The founder of the new department store was an American man by the name of Harry Gordon Selfridge, and it was this model of store and its marketing that took over the shopping experience.

You could find anything you wanted in MRA's. My figure skates, leather shoes, reversible skirts, winter boots, sweater sets, leather jackets, perfume (my first scent was Evening in Paris), toiletries, jewellery, and all my graduation gifts for high school and nursing came from here. An amethyst ring, brooch, earrings, and sterling bracelet were all gifted to me in the store's signature velvet boxes. Special occasions made for special memories. The bridal shop held magnificent gowns for the rich and famous, with designer labels and dresses for the mother of the bride and the bridal party. Silk, satin, and heavy taffeta ensembles adorned the racks. The attendant clerks were skilled in the art of fitting gowns and convincing nervous brides of their right and expensive choice.

There was a floor housing furniture, where my parents purchased my bedroom suite and later, when I married, we purchased our first set of living room furniture. The china shop, full of bright overhead lighting, was a fascinating place to see the very best in fine bone china and sterling silver, amidst beautiful crystal and decorative floral bouquets. I began to collect Royal Doulton dishes and Wallace sterling silver, even before I entered nursing.

Enough of the digression, here is the connection.

Being a student nurse was not all work and no play. Once a year our nursing school put on a large fashion show in the gymnasium, with tickets sold to those members of the public who wanted to see the latest clothing on display. It was all women's wear, and the very latest in styles and colours went on parade. The competitor to MRA's, Calp's, supplied every item in the show.

The spring fashion gala raised money for the students' recreation club. Auditions were held to select the girls who would have the honour of modelling. The successful students would then learn how to walk on the runway up the centre aisle of the auditorium.

From my diary, February 24, 1960

Tonight, I went down to try out for modelling and got chosen as one of the sixteen from seventy-five.

The most exciting part of the show was the conclusion when the bride in her wedding dress and the bridal party pranced out in all their finery. A senior student was always chosen for this, and none of us knew right away who that person would be. As a second-year student, I knew it wouldn't be me.

The following day, a note with my name on it was left at the front desk. The note read, "This is to advise you that you have been selected to model the bridal attire."

What? There's a mistake. They can't realize I'm in second year.

From my diary, February 29, 1960

I had clothes from the Grey Room, the part of the store that sold the most exclusive and expensive outfits. Probably the first and last time I'll have clothes from there. Some of what I'm wearing includes a navy-blue suit, a green shirtwaist dress, a blue silk dress and coat to match, a pink and green sports outfit. All of them are out of this world.

I knew the break in tradition would ruffle a few feathers in the senior class. Clothing consultants selected the outfits and had all of us try them on in advance of the show night.

"Miss McCarthy? We need to get your measurements for the bridal gown . . ."

The proof was in those words. I was the bride and very happy, very excited, to be chosen.

—∧ᴸ—

The day of the fashion show was a hive of activity. Vans shuttled the clothes back and forth in huge cardboard boxes that, when opened, produced a flourish of tissue paper. The outfits were hung on racks in each of the reception rooms. Each was labelled with the student's name, with the ensembles in the order they would be worn. Every room had a hairdressing station and a makeup specialist. Speed would be of the essence in the change area— removing one outfit and hastily pulling on the next, and having hair and makeup refreshed each time. Ticket holders filed in through the front doors of the residence, while the models squeezed past to the designated dressing rooms.

I saw the special bag holding the wedding gown and couldn't wait to open it; however, patience is a virtue, so it remained in the bag. The pace was quick, walking along the centre aisle with a sea of expectant faces looking up at each of us. People were making notes, and the press were snapping pictures. I loved parading around in fancy clothes and being applauded for doing so.

I wore a selection of outfits. A pillbox hat perched on my head with the linen suit. The Mediterranean cruise wear, a pink and green floral skirt and top, was enhanced by a large handbag. Bermuda shorts and a white linen blouse were a big hit, and I would be buying them afterwards. The one-piece bathing suit and sandals were on my wish list. The evening wore on, and finally, giddy with excitement, the coveted bridal outfit was taken from its clothes bag. I looked at it in wonder. And I looked again. This was not the floor-length gown of my dreams; it was knee-length.

How could they be so stupid! What bride wants to wear a short dress?

But the floor-length choice was not to be.

Fashions had changed. I modelled the knee-length, full-skirted wedding dress, and I admit I was disappointed! I wanted to feel like a princess, and instead I walked the runway with multiple petticoats picking holes in my stockings while I balanced the veil on my head. It was hard to look ethereal with my knees knocking, my hands shaking so much that petals fell from the bouquet, and my face fixed in a frozen smile. My bridesmaids entered the room ahead of me, and I glided shakily along on French-heeled leather shoes.

This might be the only time I wear a bridal dress!

After all the excitement died down, we could buy any item of clothing we wore, at cost, so I had the fun of buying a few items for future use, but the short gown went back in its bag, and we all went back to training.

Week by week, month by month, the second year of our nursing experience was ticking away in a blur of shift work and classroom time. We were young and ambitious, serious and frivolous, and all female. Naturally, we flirted and fell in and out of love. Maintaining a normal dating experience was impossible. The hours spent on shifts, and the rigid and limited number of late-night passes allowed, placed severe limits on romance.

Even so, each rotation of new interns caused a ruffle of excitement in our ranks. The men were looked over carefully. Wedding bands observed on some meant instant elimination from the possibility of a date, and the others were narrowed down by virtue of age, nationality, visiting Canada only for the duration of their studies, and other variables that played a part when scouting. All of us realized the hard life that doctors experienced with their own impossible time demands, and interns were the worst of them all, with inhumane schedules to keep. Flirtations led to romance for a few of my classmates. Some were short-lived commitments, others resulted in long-lasting marriages.

I continued to date the young man I had met in high school, but his attendance away at university didn't help us stay together. Instead, I had frequent dinner and movie dates and enjoyed the freedom of not being tied to one person. I simply was not ready.

The residence was well supervised, so if I brought a man back to sit in one of the small reception rooms, a simple moment of a kiss would likely be interrupted. The ladies at the front desk routinely glided by on their rubber-soled shoes, checking on us. While the decor of the sitting rooms was sweet, with heart-shaped pillows and comfy sofas, it was like dating in a fishbowl.

Some of my classmates were bold enough to find a way out of the residence for a late night, prying off a window screen in the basement adjacent to the back parking lot. To return the same way meant help was needed from another student, either pushing or pulling in. We only had so many after-midnight opportunities on our student card. My boldness didn't extend that far.

I met a very nice man with a head full of red hair, and we hit it off rather well. We dated, played badminton, walked the beaches, ate meals in nice restaurants, and knew that something serious was developing as time went on. It would be on-again, off-again dating, a romance that ultimately, years later, led to marriage.

In December 1961, as part of my student rotation, I was assigned to the isolation unit. It housed patients with contagious infections and undiagnosed illness. Germs spread quickly in the right environment, and isolation was the answer. I was sent to the unit for a few weeks, and since it was so close to Christmas, patients who could be discharged home were. I could count on not much to do, a nice change from the other wards where there was always a sense of too much work and too little time. The nurse in charge was a formidable person. She spent her day seated at the front desk, looking over records and charts and reading the newspaper for long stints at a time.

Each patient stayed alone in a single room. In an adjacent scrub area, staff got themselves washed, masked, and gowned in their protective uniform, then, depending on the diagnosis, added gloves.

I prepared the equipment I had to use before this protocol, then entered the patient's room and provided the treatment. Upon conclusion, the entire process went in reverse. The soiled gown, mask, and gloves were disposed of in bags and buckets, and then I washed my hands and charted the information. On to the next person and the same procedure all over again.

And so, December began to make its way to Christmas, and plans were made for the student body to take part in a carol sing on Christmas morning. Most of us would not need to look at lyrics, as the words were already in our memories. We had our collective voice, and at a set time, we were to sing together in the lobby, then make our way through the stairwells and gather on each floor. The nurses who were not getting time off formed the choir. Later, near New Year's, they would enjoy the remains of the holiday. Classmates who lived far away usually got first dibs on a few days off, including the twenty-fifth. Students who lived nearby could grab a few hours with family sometime during the season.

I was on duty on Christmas Eve, but I lived close by, so I hoped to be absent from the carols. Scheduled to work the evening shift, I walked over to the hospital as the first heavy snowflakes were drifting down. I felt a bit sorry for myself having to work that evening, as I wanted, like everyone else, to be home with family. My self-pity ended quickly when I went on duty, because the two patients remaining had long-term stays ahead of them to become well again.

I listened to the nursing report and wondered how I would spend the eight hours of the shift, given the few patients in my care. One was a middle-aged man with a leg wound that had resulted from cutting wood. It refused to heal, and after weeks of infection, the edges of the tissue gaped long and open, with the bone of the leg visible and dully gleaming. The skin had festered, and the edges were pus-coated, building up rapidly between each attempt to clean and treat. The outcome would be amputation if the infection didn't resolve. His treatment was simple: hot compresses every two hours, antibiotic powder, gauze and Teflon dressings, and rewrapping his leg. Then I took his temperature, gave him his medicines, and turned on his radio to a station playing Christmas music.

I glanced out his window. What had earlier been a few flakes was now a nor'easter, buffeting the city. A shocking amount of wind whipped the gusts in billows. Intense blowing snow coated Waterloo Street with drifts, and traffic had slowed to a crawl. St. Mary's Church looked deserted, despite the scheduled service. People were staying snug at home. My father planned to pick me up later, so I could open my gifts with him and my mother in Renforth. *Will he make it?* Safe in the hospital, the magnitude of the storm was obvious, seen but not heard.

The other patient was the same age as me, a nineteen-year-old woman who two days before had become engaged to her high school sweetheart. She had suddenly developed a very high fever and severe headache, arriving at the emergency department earlier by ambulance. The initial battery of tests done for meningitis came back negative and hadn't shown the cause of the illness. In hopes of reversing the bacteria that she was fighting, she was being vigorously treated with a powerful intravenous antibiotic. She drifted in and out of consciousness, moaning with the pain in her head.

I gave her a bed bath and sponged her body with tepid water, trying to cool her down. Her fever began a slow climb up the thermometer, alarming me when it registered 104 degrees Fahrenheit. All her medicines were administered intravenously, and I left the room, ungowned, and went to the phone to call the resident doctor. I didn't like what I heard as I stood listening at the door of her room. Her breathing was laboured and noisy. The resident arrived and we both gowned and went in to assess her again. The resident hesitated to call the patient's family doctor at home, but indecision turned to resolve, and he made the call.

In that short interval her temperature had climbed to 104.5 degrees, and her pulse had weakened. Where before she had given a slight response when asked a question, now there was none. I left the room again, came back with buckets of ice cubes and towels, and began packing them around her legs and arms, as well as across the front of her body. I stayed nearby, observing her breathing, and as the evening wore on, I monitored her fever, which held consistently too high.

The clock was ticking toward the end of my shift when the resident checked her again. Her fever had notched up even higher despite the ice and the intravenous therapy. The resident added another intravenous line to her opposite arm and infused her with a second broad spectrum antibiotic to run concurrent with the first. I had a sinking feeling that this young woman with her unknown disease might not make it.

Oh my God. She's so sick! Could she die? We don't know what she has wrong . . .

Looking out the window, the thought occurred to me that the night nurse might not make it in for duty, but a few minutes later she arrived ahead of the eleven o'clock schedule. Illuminated by the hospital lights, great walls of snow cascaded from the edge of the building and blew ferociously over everything. Again, the resident called the patient's family doctor and advised him of the status of his patient. Together they decided it was time to call her fiancé and family to the unit to be with her; sometimes the presence of family can turn a crisis around. As the great storm raged, all buses and taxis were off the roads. Even the plows had given up for a few hours, their blades no match for it. I wondered how her parents would get to the hospital in the blizzard.

I spoke with the resident. "Tell the family to get a police escort, and if we have to confirm the information, we can." I charted the evening's work for the night nurse coming on. I gave report and left the unit with a deep and bleak sense of foreboding for my young patient.

My father was an excellent driver and had assured me that he would be at the front of the residence at eleven thirty to pick me up. I waited and watched from the front door and finally saw his car lights coming up the hill, well after midnight. The car skidded and slid from side to side. He came to a final halt, quite late, but there nonetheless. We drove back home in silence, his attention fully needed to stay on the road.

In the morning, I had a few snow-filled hours at home to open presents. I helped shovel the car out and ate a great early Christmas Day dinner before my dad returned me to the hospital and the evening shift that began at 3:00 p.m. What a difference a day makes, as the saying goes. The storm had subsided, leaving great swaths of snow on the road edges. As I walked through the brightly decorated main hall, I wondered how my young woman was. I knew the answer when I stepped into the nurses' station. There was one chart in the rack, and it wasn't hers. The head nurse looked awful, and it was obvious why.

"She died, then? In the night?" I asked.

Her family and fiancé had made it to her bedside,

to sit in vigil. Planning for a wedding had been overtaken with planning her funeral. Her body was now in the morgue awaiting an autopsy. Her death at the same age as me created a painful awareness once more that life was fleeting. I still questioned whether I had chosen the right career given how hard it was to deal with loss. I stood at the door of her room, where hours before she had fought her battle. The brightness of the day bounced light off the walls, and I could almost feel her presence.

Those early lessons in life, the suffering, the loss, the unexpected surprises and shocks, all changed me in subtle ways. I was still a teenager, but now I realized the importance of living in the present moment. I began to live each day with joy and full commitment to the task, whatever it was. This budding philosophy would be reinforced over the path of my training and certainly throughout my life as it unfolded.

Chapter 10

When the second year of training ended, our black shoes and stockings were replaced with the long-desired whites, and all my classmates decided it would be a great reason to celebrate in a variety of ways. The evening before the actual whites ceremony, we gathered in rooms up and down the hallways and indulged in treats. One of the doctors sent a parcel to the front desk, a huge, fully wrapped salami from the delicatessen, along with cheese and crackers. This was a feast to us after our steady diet of ice cream floats and peanut butter sandwiches. We topped this up with a surreptitious buying of a few bottles of sherry—not wine or beer or hard liquor, but sherry. I don't know why that choice, except it might have been because of the price. We crammed into my room, took swigs of the sherry, and wolfed down the salami. From room to room, different tasty foods materialized. We ate and giggled our way through each classmate's food.

The following day we celebrated with a sumptuous banquet in the Star Lit Room at Randy's Restaurant, forty of us dressed up in pretty dresses. The broadcaster at CJCH radio dedicated a song to us, "You Don't Know What You've Got (Until You Lose It)." None of us cared about the loss of black shoes and stockings! We lined up in cars and formed a cavalcade with our black shoes tied together, dragging behind. What was it about silliness and joy that made us think everyone else should be happy? We drove around the city in a noisy, horn-honking group, screeching out songs, and the Saint John police took notice.

Sirens tend to grab your attention. We got pulled over. Briefly. They were pretty good about it when we told them what we were celebrating and why, and being young cops, they may have been fishing for a date or two. We went on our way. Later, back at the residence, we pulled on our new white shoes and stockings, paraded through the halls, and serenaded our sister students with our songs.

The following day a friend and I drove over to the Reversing Falls Bridge, a famous landmark in the city, where with every cycle of the tide, the river reverses its flow in a maelstrom of churning water. I climbed over the guardrail and down the bank, holding my old shoes and stockings in my hands. I dispatched them to a watery grave and said a permanent goodbye. Never again would I wear those tired black shoes! Cars stopped, the drivers no doubt wondering what the heck this woman was doing. The onlookers watched and waited. They may have wondered whether they were about to witness a suicide. It was soon evident that I wasn't about to do that, as I climbed back up the bank.

A lot of change happened in a single day. We posed for pictures in the hallways and front entrance, proudly showed our transformed legs, and smiled with relief to have made it to the third year. Working the first shift in white shoes and stockings, I was aware that my classmates and I were two-thirds of the way through our training. There was a new respect from the staff and doctors as they glanced at our whites; they knew what level of nursing we had achieved.

With senior student status, we pulled more shift work, and on evenings and nights the younger trainees looked to us for guidance and help. They nursed under our watchful eyes, and we finally got a taste of how our authority would evolve as we looked forward to the final months.

Our late-leave cards now noted we were seniors, and the time allowed for a late night out was 2:00 a.m., twice a month. My card was rarely used. Working so many shifts, it was not possible to take advantage of the privilege.

Change was in the air, and discussions about the role of nursing started to filter out from behind closed doors. Professional training in the future would be achieved with the choice of two streams of schooling. One option would be to obtain a university degree, and the other would be to keep the three-year diploma program in the hospital. Talk spread about uniforms, and our hard-won pride in obtaining our whites was part of the discussion. Rumours flew that in another few years the students would all enter in white dresses, no more delineation of the probie in pinstripes and the succession of bibs and caps and bar pins.

I never understood who brought these radical changes forward, but political will was about to alter the strong history of nurses' training and appearance. To my knowledge, the student body was never offered a chance to participate in these talks or to vote on whether an all-white uniform on a student was appropriate. Meanwhile, we continued our study and our work, bonding tightly together in the final months.

Soon I had to rotate to the operating room. I prepared for this by training in the classroom. Endless hours of learning about the different instruments and suture materials that would appear on the surgical trays, along with protocols for counting sponges, scrubbing, gowning—on and on it went, and all of it scared the bejeebers out of me. The trays of instruments needed in a surgical procedure filled a vast array of surfaces. There were no longer just a few items on a small tray but an entire surface covered in instruments in all sizes and shapes. The suture materials alone were intimidating enough, as the needles were not prepared in advance but had to be threaded at the time needed and required the knowledge of the appropriate thread for the task. The speed of the surgeon added to the stress of scrubbing in to assist. The pace kept the pressure on, and a slow student would suffer a sharp rebuke or a glare from the doctor. The more experience I gained, the better I became with my ability to slap an instrument into the waiting hand.

Even before I stepped foot on the hallowed floors of the operating theatre, I was shaking in my boots. Located on the seventh floor, the sickly-sweet blend of ether and nitrous oxide, in addition to the ever-present slight smell of blood from surgeries, permeated the air. I could clean it all up after an operation, but the atmosphere held its memory. While ether was used less frequently, it made its presence known throughout the operating room and wafted down through the elevator shafts to the ground floor.

There was a sense of the sacred and the vulgar in the corridors here. Some of the surgeons were crude and relieved their own tension by making disgusting jokes and comments. This was counterbalanced by the truly professional and serious nature of others. The pressures of life and death were a daily occurrence here, and it was this impending sense of what the outcome could be that permitted surgeons to vent a variety of stresses.

The patients who required an operation were brought into the hospital at least one day in advance for blood work and any preoperative tests. They stayed overnight in a hospital bed, were given a sleeping pill for a good night's rest, and were provided with a drug to prepare them for the trip to the operating theatre. They were strapped to a stretcher for the transfer and felt quite relaxed before being given a general anaesthetic.

Today's practice is vastly different. Surgery is preceded several days or weeks in advance by a pre-operative assessment in the hospital. On the day of the operation, patients come to the surgical unit at ungodly hours and wait in a large shared room where the nurses draw blood and take a history and where the anaesthetist briefly sees them. Often, depending on the scope of what is planned, the patient walks to the operating room, which contributes to a certain amount of anxiety in the few minutes before being led to the table and asked to lie down. The overnight stay of previous decades did a lot to allay fears for the patient. Today's system often means rising early and leaving home from a distance, on poor roads and possibly in bad weather.

I learned to put on a brave face when greeting patients coming into the operating room even though I was petrified that I would make a mistake. Thankfully, I never did. I had been grilled on the importance of the sterile field and taught all the implements of the trade and their variety of sizes. Retractors, scalpels and blades, scissors, forceps, syringes, Kelly forceps, needles for aspiration, different threads and catgut for suture materials—the list was long. Wearing a green cotton shift pulled over my head and tied at the waist, I learned the procedure for a surgical scrub, and I loved the ritual lathering of my hands and arms with Betadine soap, smelling of iodine and staining my skin a reddish hue. It was these moments of standing alongside the surgeon, chatting as we scrubbed, that I felt a part of the team.

I learned to gown and glove without contaminating anything by an accidental touch. I opened the sterile packs of gowns and then held one open for the surgeon to insert his arms into the sleeves while the circulating nurse tied the gown at the back. I held open the rubber gloves for the doctor, who carefully inserted his hands inside while I pulled them above the arm cuff of the gown with a snap.

We wore operating room caps that squished our

hair down so not a strand peeked out, and masks covered our nose and mouth so all that showed were our eyes. In the absence of other visible facial features, eyes took on a new intensity. We wore shoe covers to protect our feet from the inevitable blood and fluid splatters and to avoid contaminating the operating theatre. Dressed as we were, indistinguishable and nearly sterile, we were an early cotton version of today's haz-mat outfit.

The time came for me to assist in the small operating room where tonsillectomies were performed. I had wretched childhood memories of my own surgery, the rubber mask clamping down on my face, the reek of ether, and the state of light unconsciousness sounding in my ears like a train roaring through. As I proceeded to help the surgeon extract the tonsils from a little boy, the recollection flashed in my brain of waking up in a high-sided bed, alone and crying, blood dripping down my chin. These were considered minor operations but still had the risk of hemorrhage. I was happy to complete that experience, which was always quick and bloody, and move on to larger and more complicated surgeries.

I prepared the instrument table after the circulating nurse removed the draped linen cover, and I carefully and accurately counted each piece of metal, all cross-referenced to the written record kept by the non-scrubbed nurse. Together we counted every gauze sponge in every package, for God forbid that, at the end of the operation when the final tally was recorded, a sponge be missing or an instrument be unaccounted for. Needles and thread packages received the same routine, and if excess bleeding used up all the sponges, the counting and cross-referencing recurred with each new package of gauze squares opened. The tiniest gauze squares were called peanuts, and they were the easiest to lose. My classmate Donna recalls frantically crawling on her hands and knees under the operating room table looking for a lost peanut, while the surgeon, looming above, closed the incision. No pressure!

When all was ready, the patient would be rolled on a stretcher into the operating theatre and partly sedated, then transferred over to the bed to be positioned and draped with the initial linen covers. The tension in the room magnified with the entrance of the surgeon and the team of resident and intern. The anaesthetist would begin his vital role of sedating and anaesthetizing the person. Once that was done, the final surgical drapes were positioned, and the nod was given for the surgeon to proceed.

My role was to hand over the instruments, quickly answering the demand for this and that, using the right pressure to slap it into his hand. I first passed the scalpel and blade for the initial cut into the skin, followed by the doctor making a careful incision down through the layers. A lot of blood was lost in surgery, so Kelly forceps were clipped onto large bleeders. Square sponges and tiny peanuts were used, and small bleeders were cauterized with the accompanying smell of burned tissue. The sponges were quickly used up, more packages were opened and counted, while the work went on.

The four-by-four-inch gauze pads were folded in a special way and clipped to forceps, used to dab the blood while the suction machine sucked up the excess bleeding into a glass jar. The pressure felt intense, answering demands, gathering specimens, counting old and new sponges, recounting, preparing sutures, all the while listening to the demands of the surgeon and slapping instruments into his outstretched hand with just the right intensity. Occasionally, I would have such adrenalin flowing that I would use too much force, slapping the palm of the doctor with a resounding thwack. This would be met with a reproachful glance. The resident or intern was also under pressure and made demands. The discarded and bloodied sponges were tossed into a bucket and had to be counted before they were disposed of.

I never felt confident about the suture materials. No matter how often I prepared them and threaded the different needles, my stress made me feel uncertain about what to use when. While I knew the book work, I felt so afraid of handing off the wrong threaded needle. Sometimes the surgeons sensed this and reached across the tray to select what they wanted, but most of the time I was able to respond properly.

Once the close-up procedure began, the rapid pace of rechecking the instrument and sponge count intensified, as no one wanted to be the one to say there was a sponge missing or a Kelly forcep not accounted for and then assumed to be inside the patient. In one of the rare instances of hitting the panic button, an abdominal retractor was noted to be missing one of its screws. Hell hath no fury like a doctor looking for a screw while the student frantically inspected everything on the table that had passed through her hands. Finally, X-ray was called, and the screw was found inside the abdomen—thank God, before closure.

The circulating nurse prepared the specimens removed from the patient while I finalized the undraping and removal of bloodied linens.

The unconscious person was transferred to a waiting stretcher and moved to the recovery room while students cleaned up the theatre. Linens were stripped and bagged for the laundry, the tables were meticulously scrubbed down, blood spills were washed from anything and everything, the floors were mopped and rinsed, and the operating table was reset. We removed the used and bloodied instruments to the soiled utility room, where we washed and dried them and reset the instrument trays before bundling and labelling them to be sent for sterilization. Quite the routine!

The operating rooms were checked for all supplies, and everything was topped up to the requisite number of gowns and gloves. At each nursing shift, all stainless-steel tables and containers were wiped down, and everything would be ready. The student's job meant being on one's feet for the entire shift of eight hours.

At the end of the day, we trudged back to the residence to shower and change, then to collapse on our beds and chat with other students and friends. Some of us were on call. The dreaded words none of us wanted to hear were "Phone call from the operating room supervisor," meaning an emergency surgery was about to happen. We would hurriedly re-dress and take ourselves back to the hospital and scrub again for set-up. I do not recall many of the sixty-one operations that I scrubbed in for, but I do recall the most shocking one.

First, there is a story to tell that reconnects me with my teenage years growing up in Renforth and around Saint John. The port city had its seamier side in the streets adjacent to the waterfront, and every port had its "house of ill repute." There was street prostitution, but most of it was contained to the brothels. As silly teenagers we drove our parents' cars through the red-light district and honked the horns at the prostitutes who sat in the window, their breasts exposed, hands beckoning to passersby and a distinct red lamp casting its glow. If anyone had ever recognized my dad's car cruising past a whorehouse, I shudder to think what would have resulted. Why we thought this was fun eludes me, but we would often, on a dare, drive back and forth and toot the horn, cruising along after dark.

The brothel had the advantage of offering safety in numbers. It never entered my head to wonder about the young women and how they had come to their trade. It didn't occur to me that there was risk for sex workers, such was my ignorance. Whorehouses were accepted in the port, as a fact of life and a sexual service industry.

My lack of conscious awareness was about to change. I was on call for the evening shift in the operating room, as students had to take their turn to scrub in in case of an emergency. I received the call from the switchboard that I was required. With a sense of urgency, I dressed and dashed. Arriving in the OR in record time, I hurried into the green shapeless uniform and went to the sink to prep my hands and arms with soap and a brush. The supervisor came over to me and without explanation advised me that I was to stand by if needed and that I wasn't to enter the operating room at all.

Certainly, it was strange to be called over, ready to go, and not be put to immediate use. I looked through the glass window and observed a young girl on the stretcher, lit by the bright glare of overhead lights. I was told she was a seventeen-year-old prostitute, brought in by ambulance from the brothel. I would never know what pain she had endured before the madam running the place gave in to her cries for help and called the ambulance team. She burned with a high fever and lay on the table, sedated. Her huge, distended abdomen swelled under the drapery. The decision to keep the staff in the room to a bare minimum had been made because no one knew exactly what was wrong with her, and the risk of infection was great.

I continued to peer through the window as the surgeon placed the scalpel blade on her exposed skin and made the first cut. Pus shot out of her with intense force and hit the overhead spotlight, dripping back on the open wound, and showering the surgical team. She had sepsis from infection and pelvic disease, with an abdomen full of virulent bacteria. It was overwhelming and required the table drapes to be changed, while the entire scrubbed team had to gown again. One circulating nurse couldn't do it all by herself. My standby status quickly changed, and I was ordered to get in there fast. The supervisor held the swing door open for me and I joined the effort to save the young girl's life. Ultimately, she was gone beyond any ability of surgical intervention, as the infection had clearly consumed her insides. She died after surgery, a young woman whose life as a prostitute had been painfully short, ending in more pain and an early death. I chose never to childishly drive through the brothel district again.

Serving in the OR was followed by a rotation in the recovery room. There was no electronic monitoring, and the student, under the supervision of the registered nurse in charge, closely kept watch over the unconscious patient. Everyone came from their operation with an intratracheal tube inserted down the throat, keeping the airway open and preventing the swallowing of the tongue.

We checked skin colour, blood pressure, pulse, the rate of respiration, and the dressing covering the surgical incision every fifteen minutes. Out of the depths of being unconscious, the patient would slowly and groggily come to semi-consciousness, gagging on the tube in the throat. Awakening was a slow process, but once eyes opened and the tube was being retched up, I would remove it and commence some limited conversation to make sure they were staying groggily alert. Everyone groaned with pain, while moans, cries, and vomiting were common. Injections of narcotics were given. Although surgeries were performed with the patient not having had any food, the anaesthetic often triggered the heaves. The intravenous bags were changed as much as needed, blood transfusions were given, and I went back and forth to each patient, logging all the vitals and almost enjoying every minute. It was so different from ward experience, and in the brief moments of not pumping up blood pressure cuffs, I would sit at the desk rolling up bandages and doing chores. The recovery room was a short-term experience, and I never heard anyone complain about it.

It is hard to say where the final year went. We steadily carried on, learning more from experience now than in the classroom, and we took on greater responsibilities over the younger students. Soon to be placed on our cap was the "black band," the tiny, thin strip of velvet ribbon that would be attached to our caps with a stitch at either end. This single piece of ribbon really said it all. The end was in sight, we were ready to graduate, and we had made it through all the challenges of the training period. Our director of nursing handed out the bands, and I know she took pride in doing so. Here were "her nurses." Each of us happily attached the band to our caps, and after looking in the mirror many times, I got used to the image peering back. Almost there! The first time on the wards with a black ribbon on my cap, I was congratulated by senior staff and met with respectful glances from those around. The younger students looked on too, knowing their important day would come.

My graduation dance was coming up fast, and I had no date. Panic was about to set in, when someone suggested I ask one of the interns who didn't have a girlfriend. I approached him on the wards to see if he would take me to the event and at least give me the semblance of a partner to celebrate with. To my surprise, he was pleasant enough and said yes, so I began the search for a nice dress to wear.

The Symphony of Fashion was held at the Admiral Beatty Hotel, an elegant show in the Georgian ballroom showcasing the latest and most expensive clothing for the city's families with high disposable incomes. Mrs. Arthur L. Irving modelled a floor-length white gown in heavy heirloom taffeta with large blue roses and green leaves. It was a Nina Ricci design with deep folds of fabric and a bouffant effect at the hip. It had a fitted top and narrow straps and looked splendid on Mrs. Irving. I knew when I saw the picture of it in the newspaper, I had to have it as my own. The gown was being sold at Calp's, and I went in the next day with my mother, and she agreed to buy it for a small fortune. It fit me like it had been custom made for my frame, so I was all set! Our dance would be held the night after graduation, so at least I was ready.

Our commencement exercises were held at the Saint John High School auditorium on Thursday evening, June 7, 1962. I had my hair set and made sure I had a freshly laundered and starched uniform to wear, along with a fresh cap. I posed for pictures with a beautiful bouquet of a dozen red roses, and to this day when I see pictures of myself, glowingly proud in the moment, I wonder how I had such a tiny waistline, accented by the band of the apron.

I think all my classmates looked their stunning best on that day.

We gathered at the auditorium, and the evening began with a rousing rendition of the national anthem. The opening prayer was spoken by the Reverend H. G. Taylor, followed by the chairman of the board of the Saint John General Hospital, Dr. Carl Trask, who gave his comments. For the last time, we stood as a class and spoke the words of the Nightingale pledge before the assembly. Next, our navy-blue leather-bound diplomas were presented by Senator Clarence Emerson, followed by the big moment when each of us received our fourteen-karat gold pins. Our director pinned each of us, one by one placing the distinctive medal over our hearts, as we grinned away. My mom and dad were dressed up in their finest, smiling happily at me from their seats near the front. This was the moment that three years of hard work and study had brought us to. Our lives were changing and soon we would no longer be part of a class of students. We would be looking for a job. With a real paycheque.

Senator Emerson gave the address, and to be truthful, I don't recall a single word he said. There were prizes to be given out, for some of my class-mates were going on for further study. Marilyn Bates gave the valedictory address. She was wonderful and reminded us that we were the largest class in the history of the General.

During her remarks, Marilyn said, "Progress is not made by standing still, so we must now break our family circle as we venture into the battle of life. We shall meet with much turmoil and confusion but equipped with the philosophy for good living and the lessons of citizenship, sportsmanship, and relationships that we have learned at the Saint John General Hospital School of Nursing, we should be able to withstand the obstacles."

Family and friends celebrated with us into the evening. My doctor date turned out to be a lot of fun. He provided the customary corsage worn at my wrist and picked me up in his car to go to the ballroom at the Admiral Beatty Hotel. We had received printed invitations to the dinner and dance, held by the alumnae association. The meal seemed to take forever, and most of us were not that interested in food, with the ever-present concern that our beautiful dresses might get soiled before we were ever on the dance floor! The music was live, and the hits of the day were played. My date turned out to be an exceptional dancer, so we were up for every tune of the night, with my gorgeous dress an instant hit. My hair was swept up in a French twist, and I truly felt like a princess.

Friends gathered in one of the rooms afterwards and the hours slipped away as we sipped champagne and generally made the wonderful memories of a lifetime. Cinderella left her ball at the stroke of midnight; we left mine closer to 2:00 a.m., to return to the residence. To bed, nurse princess, to sleep and dream.

We crammed for exams and wrote them, all of us fearing failure and hoping that we would get through the final hurdle and receive our registered nurse distinction. And guess what? We all did. One moment we were students, and the next, we were looking for jobs and moving from the residence.

Nursing practice was studied in all three years of our lectures, building layer upon layer of knowledge so that we could function on the medical floors with their life-and-death scenarios. Over the first two years, 586 hours of lecture time and 134 hours of lab time were achieved; a total of 978 days of nursing practice were accumulated by the end of the three-year program.

In writing this memoir, I am profoundly aware that the years of professional training made me a competent, focused, pragmatic thinker. This stood me in good stead as I pursued my career, becoming the night supervisor in obstetrics at the Saint John General Hospital, after I completed my diploma in obstetrics and gynecology at the Margaret Hague Maternity Hospital in Jersey City, New Jersey. I also worked as the head nurse in the postpartum unit in the Grace Maternity Hospital in Halifax, Nova Scotia. I retired from nursing after my two daughters were born and later became politically active. I was elected first as a Halifax County councillor in 1976, then became the first mayor of the town of Bedford, NS. I later became the president of the Nova Scotia Advisory Council on the Status of Women, followed by my appointment as the executive director of the Nova Scotia Liberal Party. In 1993, I was elected to the provincial legislature and was appointed party whip, then deputy speaker of the assembly. In my second election, I was appointed to the executive council of government, serving as the minister for community services, minister of the civil service, minister responsible for the Disabled Persons Commission, and minister responsible for the Status of Women Act. I credit nursing for all it enabled me to do throughout my lifetime.

Epilogue

BY 1967, DEPARTMENTS OF UROLOGY AND OPH-thalmology were much needed and became integrated into the Saint John General Hospital. This was followed in 1972 by a rheumatic disease unit, and in 1973, a special neonatal care unit was established.

The decision to move nursing education to a university setting ultimately caused the demise of the in-hospital school. The last class graduated from the Saint John General Hospital School of Nursing in 1972. The General closed its doors to training, and in 1982, the hospital itself closed, replaced by the new regional hospital in the western end of the city. Political decisions rest in the hands of the few; those who are elected can make profound and far-reaching decisions behind closed doors, in meeting rooms and cabinet rooms. Thus, the fate of the Saint John General Hospital was decided. The General emptied its rooms, and its use ended forever.

The hospital was boarded up and abandoned to

rats, pigeons, and vagrants. Its corridors became wandering grounds for druggies and vandals, who would set the occasional fire for warmth at night. Without the aid of a watchman or an alarm system, the destruction became so complete that no return to any function was possible. In one incident, youths entered the building, walked up the stairs to the eighth floor, and tossed steel lockers out of smashed windows. Teens looking for adventure wandered unopposed through the winding and dark corridors. The lights were out, literally, and the hospital sat forlorn, with its memories trapped inside.

I had an opportunity to tour the building at a nursing reunion. Those of us who dared, visited, and stepped through the debris of the corridors. For the last time, our footsteps walked the hallways.

What a mess.

Who could do this?

Why isn't the city securing the building?

Sadness and tears welled up in me as I looked at the curling floor tiles in the hallways, the desecrated operating theatres, the smashed windows, and the permeating odour of urine and feces left behind by vagrants. Peeling paint, cracked wall tiles, and the presence of memories past were not about to save the structure.

Recollections filled my brain.

I drowned in the waters of the past with every

step through the ripped-apart spaces. We all knew this was the death knell for the building and that city council must act before someone died inside. As I wandered through, looking in rooms where the old man with asthma scared me to death, the young woman with cancer had died as I started to feed her, and the patient in infectious diseases had passed in the night, the operating room with its drama and fearsome experiences, the case room and its life-and-death moments, including the tiny conceptus in a bowl, its heart stopping while I baptized it, I felt that a lifetime of emotional marks had been engraved on my spirit in just three years of training.

The hospital had many hopeless iterations of use, and all came to naught. It had become "the yellow brick elephant," according to newspaper columnist Gerry Maher, and it would cost an estimated $1 million a year to merely maintain it as an empty edifice while reviews were conducted as to what to potentially do with the building. City councillors struggled with the issue; it was determined that it would cost $2 million to take the building down. Meanwhile, the nurses' residence was demolished at a cost of $130,000. While historians reacted, and former patients pensively recalled their time spent in hospital, the decision was made to implode the structure.

A hospital is woven together from many things. Bricks, tile, glass, metal—all a glorious architectural monument. On the day of the implosion, it was featherweight against the force of dynamite.

On December 10, 1995, the General Hospital was imploded, observed by thousands of spectators, kept back at a safe distance. The huge fortress on the hill, a landmark for decades, was gone. The brick-and-mortar structure blew inward, and the cloud of dust rose overhead; it was all over in seconds. The majestic dome, visited by me as a student, refused to break apart, however, and down it came, finally settling on the mass of rubble, while a great sigh went up from the crowd. The implosion can be viewed on YouTube, and it is worth a look.

The *Saint John Times Globe* of December 11, 1995, quoted William Butler Yeats in its story about the demolition: "All changed, changed utterly: A terrible beauty is born."

The Irving empire generously moved the dome to a new location and erected it on a structure to become a tourist attraction. It also became a place of poignant memories for the nurses who would gather at reunion times, visit the dome, and stand in front of the display, each nurse with her own thoughts of her own time.

Today's hospitals are noisy and tense. The atmosphere in the units is focused on technology and computer charting, and the lack of a recognizable nursing uniform contributes hugely to the overall change. Gone are the white uniforms and caps, replaced by colourful and ill-fitting scrubs. Gone are the polished and shining bright white shoes, replaced by sneakers of all colours. One cannot tell the cleaning staff from the professional staff in many locales, except for the presence of a stethoscope slung around the neck. The strict no-jewellery policy is gone, and various hair lengths and styles have replaced the standard short hair off the collar. I believe professional appearance lost the battle, and I profess my bias. We looked more like nurses back then.

Today's nurses face a tremendous challenge, with too few of them to meet the changing demands of the times. Government restrictions on the numbers of entrants into the profession have created a chronic shortage of staff, and huge demands for overtime hours have added to the heavy load of twelve-hour shifts. The COVID-19 pandemic added to the existing burdens of the profession, and as always, registered nurses stepped up to the plate to answer the call. All nurses know the cost on themselves and their families, and yet they continue to do the job with resilience and skill. To all of you who serve, thank you and God Bless!

SAINT JOHN GENERAL HOSPITAL
SCHOOL OF NURSING
SAINT JOHN, N. B.

M. JANE STEPHENSON, R.N.
Director of Nursing

July 24, 1959.

Miss Francene J. McCarthy,
Burton Brae, Renforth, N.B.

Dear Miss McCarthy:

Your application for admission to this School of Nursing has been accepted. The class will assemble on Monday, September 7th, 1959. Please report to the Nurses Residence not later than 8 p.m. on that day. I am enclosing a measurement chart for your uniforms, which is to be filled out and sent to Bland & Company, Montreal, together with cheque to cover the amount. Please take care of this at once so that your uniforms will be delivered to the hospital in time.

It will be necessary for you to bring with you: -
1. Two pairs of black leather oxfords, leather heels of military height, with rubber lifts.
2. Black nylon stockings.
3. Watch with second hand, not necessarily a wrist-watch.
4. Housecoat with slippers, - soft moccasin type.
5. Two face cloths.
6. $25.00 which will provide for Student Association fee, both local and provincial organizations; 1st year: National League of Nursing Education Achievement Test fee; closet and room key; 3rd year: New Brunswick Association of Registered Nurses examination fee. Please note that, if for any reason you do not remain in the school, this money will not be refunded.

Since closet space in the Residence is somewhat limited, you are asked to bring as little luggage as possible. Much of your time will be spent in uniform or a housecoat, so you will not need as many clothes as you have previously. Because you will be wearing bibs and aprons you will probably feel a slip is unnecessary on duty. Luggage should be addressed to the Nurses' Residence, Waterloo Street, Saint John.

Students are permitted to sleep out of residence on the night before their day off, or, if their hours are from 7 to 10 the following morning. Please return written consent of your parents to your sleeping out of residence at these times, also, for leaving residence at 11:30 p.m. if on evening duty, to remain out overnight with parents, relatives, or friends. Authorization permit must also be submitted for the administration of B.C.G. and Salk Poliomyelitis vaccine.

I hope that you will enjoy your three years in our School of Nursing and derive much personal, as well as professional satisfaction from your chosen work. The interest and promise of effort you have already shown through our correspondence, if continued at a high level, will be richly rewarding.

Please write immediately, confirming your intention to enter the September class.

Yours sincerely,

M. Jane Stephenson,
Director of Nursing.

MJS:HM.

Saint John General Hospital School of Nursing acceptance letter

Clothing list for Nurses' Residence at Saint John General Hospital

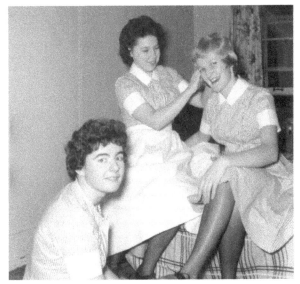

Helpful friends

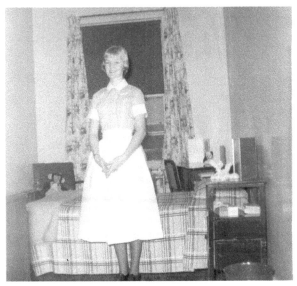

Proud probie, September 1959

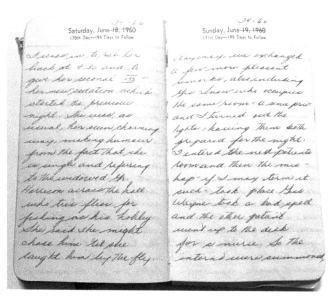

Nursing pay stub

Pages from my diary

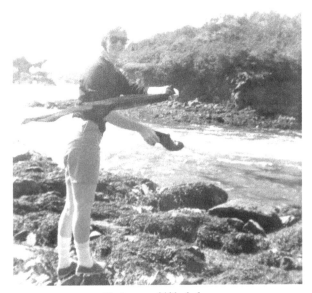

Tossing my old black shoes

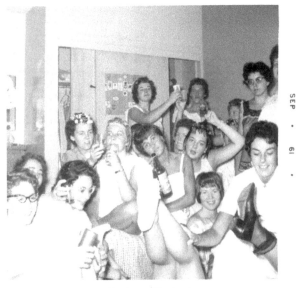

Senior whites party

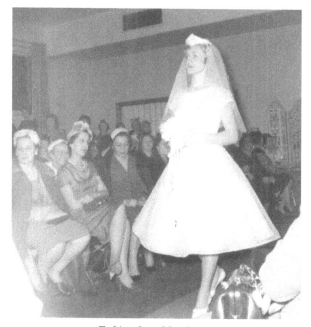

Fashion show, March 1960

T32 2M-10-60   S E N I O R

SAINT JOHN GENERAL HOSPITAL
TRAINING SCHOOL FOR NURSES

2 A.M.   LATE LEAVE CARD

Month   March to August

Name   Francene McCarthy

Class   S e n i o r

2 LATE LEAVES

March   April   May   June

SLEEP OUTS   August

Late Leave Card

Francene Cosman

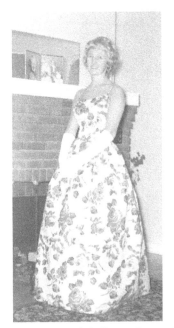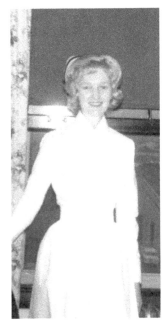

Left: ballgown, Sept. 1962; Right: with black band

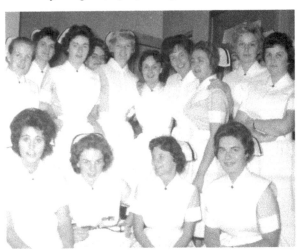

Nursing class

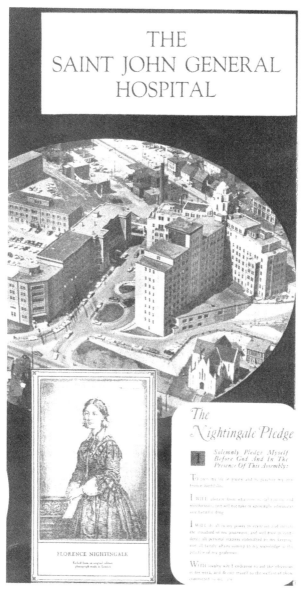

The Nightingale Pledge

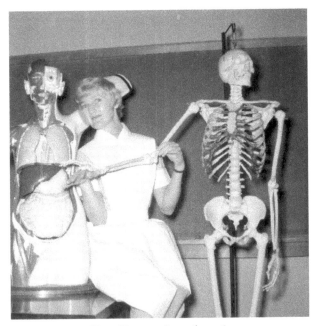

Nurse Francene, September 1962

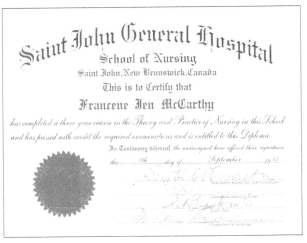

School of Nursing Diploma

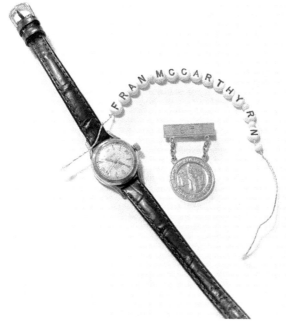

Watch and jewellery

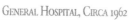

General Hospital, Circa 1962

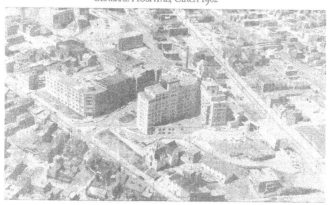

Saint John General Hospital, c.1962

Appendix 1: The Florence Nightingale Pledge

"I solemnly pledge myself before God and in the presence of this assembly, to pass my life in purity and to practice my profession faithfully. I will abstain from whatever is deleterious and mischievous, and will not take or administer any harmful drug. I will do all in my power to elevate the standard of my profession, and will hold in confidence all personal matters committed to my keeping, and all family affairs coming to my knowledge in the practice of my calling. With loyalty will I endeavour to aid the physician in his work, and devote myself to the welfare of those committed to my care."

I thought the pledge had been written by the founder of modern nursing, Florence Nightingale, herself. It was not. It was named to honour her work but was composed in 1893 by Lystra Gretter, an instructor of nursing at the old Harper Hospital in Detroit, Michigan.

Appendix 2: Songs We Sang

"A Moment of Song" (to the tune of "Memories")
Training days, training days
Days of joy and pain
When we worked and sometimes shirked
Seeking future gain.
Rules to learn, we dared not spurn
Nursing cares and ways
Though today we are grads
Yet our memory still lags
When we think of our training days.

(Tune: "My Bonnie Lies Over the Ocean")
The years of probation are over
We're graduate nurses at last
We're sporting black bands on our headgear
For the days of training are past.
(Chorus): Glad days, sad days
The days of our training are gone
Gay days, grey days
The days of our training are gone
So everyone join in the chorus
And sing like the birds in the trees
Though nightingales aren't always nurses,
Every nurse must a Nightingale be.

Appendix 3: Poems from Yearbook of 1962

A Nurse's Prayer

written by Francene Cosman

Dear Father,
Grant me a smile for the faint-hearted and weak, that they
may take courage at the receiving of such a gift.
Grant me gentle hands with which to soothe away
the tears
of pain and endless hours of suffering.
Grant me the sense to know how to help a man, not with
Meaningless trivialities, but with heart-to-
heart communication.
Grant me quiet ways so that I may enter a room
and, finding
peace within, I may leave without disturbing it.
Finally, Father, grant me a sound mind in a healthy body
To do your work in the best way possible.

Inspirations
written by Carol Reid

Inspirations come and go
And if unheeded
They pass into oblivion
Never to return
Except to haunt the heart,
Which knows
That opportunity has
Passed the port,
Which might have harboured
A great ship.

Glossary

Amniotic sac - the fluid-filled sac that contains and protects a fetus in the womb.

Anus - the lower end of the rectum which exits the body.

Bleeders - the small blood vessels that would normally stop losing blood on their own but didn't during surgery and thus had to have the intervention of small metal forceps before being tied off with a suture.

Cautery - using an instrument to burn a blood vessel to stop it from bleeding.

Carbolic soap - a mildly antiseptic soap containing carbolic acid.

Cleft palate - a narrow opening along the roof of the mouth. In a severe case this can extend into the upper lip.

Colostrum - the first secretion of pre-milk after giving birth. It is rich in antibodies that provide protection to newborns.

Cyanosed - a bluish discolouration of the skin and mouth resulting from not enough oxygen circulating in the blood.

Enema - injection of fluids into the rectum to cleanse or stimulate the emptying of its contents.

Episiotomy - a surgical cut made in the perineum during childbirth.

Fontanelle - the soft spots on an infant's head where the bony plates that make up the skull have not yet come together.

Fundus - the upper part of the uterus.

Hydrocephalic - an abnormal buildup of fluid deep within the brain, causing swelling and putting pressure on the tissues of the brain.

Intratracheal - within the trachea of the throat where a plastic tube can be inserted to maintain breathing.

Meconium - the first poop of the newborn which can also happen before birth, signifying distress in the fetus prior to birth.

Microcephalic - a condition where a baby's head is much smaller than expected due to lack of proper brain growth.

Mid forceps - the use of forceps during delivery when the fetal head is coming down the vagina but is not able to progress to birth.

Nitrous oxide - a colourless gas commonly used for sedation and pain relief.

Perineum - the muscular area between the vagina and the anus.

Rigor mortis - after-death change resulting in the stiffening of the body muscles.

Sepsis - the body's extreme response to an infection.

Transverse - the position where the baby's head is on one side of the mother's body and the feet on the other, rather than being in the head-down position.

Triage - assigning the degree of urgency to wounds or illness to decide the order of treatment.

Urethra - the tube that allows urine to pass out of the body.

Vascular bed - the network of blood vessels throughout the body.

About the Author

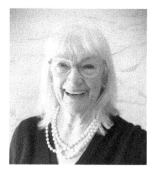

Emerging from a challenging and dysfunctional early childhood, Francene was determined to be strong and achieve goals that included continuing education and a career. She chose nursing and entered the three-year program at the Saint John General Hospital in New Brunswick. After graduation in 1962, she enrolled in a six-month post grad at the Margaret Hague Hospital in Jersey City, New Jersey, across from the lights of Manhattan. Her social conscience was awakened, and she participated in the black civil rights movement, joining in marches to support the cause of freedom and equality. At the age of twenty-two, she returned to New Brunswick and became the night supervisor of the obstetrical service (the delivery rooms), post-partum floor and the nursery of the Saint John General Hospital. Later, marriage took her to Fredericton and the Victoria Public Hospital, where she worked in the case room. Following a move to Nova Scotia, she worked in the former Grace Maternity Hospital in the case room, and later became the head nurse on the post-partum floor. After the birth of her second daughter, she retired.

Nursing provided strong foundational skills that underpinned future political involvement. A long political career ensued, first as a county councillor, then the first mayor of Bedford, NS. She was appointed president of the provincial Status of Women; four years later she chaired the task force on the concerns of women and became the executive director of the Liberal Party. In 1993, she was elected to the NS Legislature and became deputy speaker. In her second term of office, she was appointed to Executive Council as Minister of Community Services, Minister for the Civil Service and Minister of the Status of Women. She served six years on the board of governors of the Art Gallery of Nova Scotia.

She currently is the curator of the Scott Manor House in Bedford, enjoys painting, and still speaks out on community issues.

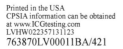

Printed in the USA
CPSIA information can be obtained
at www.ICGtesting.com
LVHW022357131123
763870LV00011BA/421